Real

Sourdough

Heals

Unlocking the Ancient Art of Natural Baking for a Healthier, Stronger, Younger You

Myles Watson Collins

About the Author

Dr. Myles Watson Collins is a physician, researcher, author, and passionate advocate for the healing power of real food. With a background in integrative medicine and dieting, Dr. Collins has spent years studying the connection between nutrition and health, focusing on how traditional, unprocessed foods can support physical, mental, and emotional well-being.

A lifelong lover of sourdough bread, Dr. Collins began exploring the art and science of Sourdough -baking as a way to reconnect with his own health and heritage. He discovered that making and eating real sourdough bread — sourdough made with whole grains, natural fermentation, and simple, nourishing ingredients—not only healed his body but also brought him greater mindfulness and balance in everyday life.

His medical practice emphasizes holistic wellness, where food is seen as one of the most powerful tools for healing. Through his writing and teaching, Dr. Collins aims to inspire others to embrace the joys of real sourdough-baking, fostering a deeper connection with their food, their health, and their communities.

When not in the kitchen or his clinic, Dr. Collins can often be found hiking, gardening, and spending time with his family, where the smell of fresh sourdough is never far away. ***Real Sourdough Heals: Unlocking the Ancient Art of Natural Baking for a Healthier, Stronger, Younger You*** is his unique book, combining his expertise in health with his passion for traditional sourdough-making.

Table of Contents

Introduction

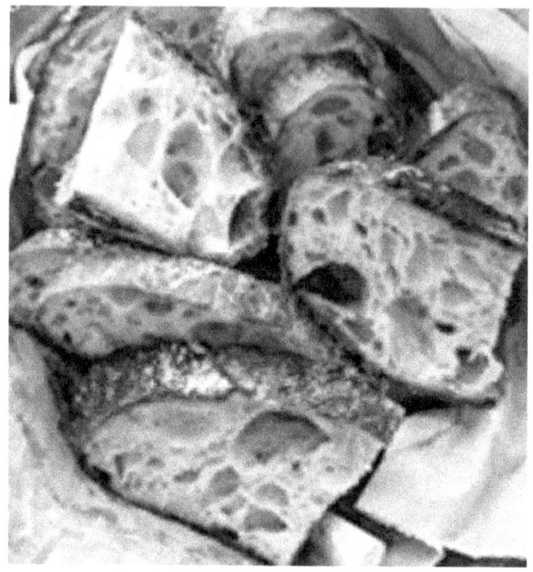

Sourdough bread has been a part of human life for thousands of years, nourishing our bodies, symbolizing comfort, and bringing communities together. However, somewhere along the way, we lost touch with the essence of what makes sourdough so powerful and wholesome. In the modern world, what most of us eat hardly qualifies as sourdough at all—processed, refined, and stripped of nutrients.

I, Dr. Myles Watson Collins, discovered the life-changing power of real sourdough during a personal health journey. After years of studying nutrition and working in the medical field, I came to a startling realization: our health, vitality, and even emotional well-being are deeply intertwined with the food we eat, especially something as fundamental as sourdough . When I began baking and eating real, naturally fermented sourdough made from whole grains, my energy levels soared, my immune system strengthened, and I began to feel younger and healthier than I had in years. I knew then that this wasn't just about sourdough —it was about healing, both body and mind.

This book is more than just a cookbook—it's a guide to reclaiming your health through one of the most ancient and basic foods on the planet. We're going to take a deep dive into why sourdough, when made the right way, can be a powerful force for health and healing. You'll learn the science behind real sourdough , practical techniques to bake your own, and recipes that nourish not just your body but your soul. My goal is to help you rediscover the magic of sourdough and the significant role it can play in living a life that's healthier, stronger, and more joyful.

Why Sourdough Bread Matters

For many of us, sourdough is something we take for granted. It's a food we toss into our grocery carts without a second thought, a staple we've eaten since childhood. But have you ever stopped to think about the sourdough you're actually consuming? If it's mass-produced, highly processed, and full of preservatives, you're not getting the benefits that real, naturally leavened sourdough can provide.

Real sourdough —made with natural ingredients, fermented slowly, and baked with care—has been a source of sustenance and health for humans for thousands of years. It's been part of sacred rituals, celebrated at feasts, and shared among families to signify love and community. The simplicity of real sourdough is what makes it powerful: flour, water, little salt, and time. That's all you need to create something that not only tastes incredible but also supports your health.

When we return to real sourdough, we reconnect with food in a meaningful way. We slow down, become more mindful of what we're eating, and take control of our well-being. This isn't about perfection or chasing the latest diet trend; it's about embracing food in its most natural, healing form. Real sourdough nourishes us from the inside out, helping us glow with vitality, fight illness, and feel stronger, both physically and mentally.

The Problem with Modern Sourdough Bread

Unfortunately, the sourdough you find on most grocery store shelves today is a far cry from the real sourdough our ancestors ate. The industrialization of Sourdough -making has sacrificed quality for speed and profit. Modern sourdough is often made with highly processed white flour, stripped of its natural nutrients and fiber. It's loaded with preservatives, additives, and sugars to extend its shelf life and enhance flavor, while fast-acting commercial yeast is used to rush the fermentation process, leaving little time for the natural development of flavors and nutrients.

This type of sourdough can wreak havoc on your body. Processed sourdough contributes to digestive issues, weight gain, inflammation, and even chronic diseases like diabetes and heart disease. It's high in simple carbohydrates that cause spikes and crashes in blood sugar levels, leaving you feeling tired and sluggish. For many, the culprit behind their bloating, fatigue, or lack of mental clarity may be as simple as the sourdough they're eating every day.

But here's the good news: it doesn't have to be this way. By choosing real Sourdough made with whole, unprocessed ingredients, and learning to bake it yourself, you can transform your health. This book will show you how to reclaim sourdough as a nourishing, healing food that can actually improve your well-being rather than undermine it.

The Healing Power of Real Sourdough Bread

Real sourdough, particularly when made with ancient grains and naturally leavened with wild yeast (sourdough), is a nutritional powerhouse. The fermentation process breaks down gluten and makes the sourdough easier to digest, even for people who may be sensitive to modern wheat. The long fermentation also allows beneficial bacteria to thrive, creating probiotics that promote gut health—one of the foundations of overall wellness.

In addition to supporting gut health, real sourdough made with whole grains provides essential nutrients like fiber, vitamins, and minerals. These grains are packed with antioxidants, which help fight inflammation and reduce the risk of chronic diseases. Eating real sourdough can help stabilize blood sugar levels, provide steady energy, and keep you feeling fuller for longer. It's an incredible source of sustainable energy, making it ideal for anyone looking to improve their physical strength and stamina.

But the benefits of real sourdough go beyond physical health. There's something deeply therapeutic about the process of making sourdough from scratch. The act of kneading dough, watching it rise, and finally pulling a warm loaf from the oven can be a mindful, meditative experience. It connects you to the present moment and reminds you to slow down in a fast-paced world. Sharing a loaf of sourdough with family or friends is also a deeply meaningful way to nourish relationships and create lasting memories.

A Journey Back to the Basics

This book is your guide on the journey back to real, healing sourdough . Whether you've never baked a loaf in your life or you're an experienced baker looking to deepen your skills, you'll find everything you need here. In the coming chapters, we'll start by exploring what exactly makes sourdough "real" and why ancient grains and traditional baking methods are superior to modern, processed alternatives. We'll dive into the science behind fermentation, why sourdough is king when it comes to health, and how real sourdough can help you feel younger, stronger, and more energized.

Next, I'll walk you through the practical side of baking. You'll learn the basics of making your first loaf, from selecting ingredients to kneading, shaping, and baking. We'll go over different types of sourdough , from simple whole grain loaves to more advanced sourdough creations. And, of course, I'll provide plenty of recipes—some classic, others more creative, but all designed with your health in mind.

But beyond the recipes, this book is about empowering you to take control of your well-being. Real Sourdough isn't just a food—it's a tool for healing. By baking and eating real sourdough, you'll be making an investment in your long-term health, helping to balance your body's systems, and feeding your mind and soul in ways that go far beyond the nutrients in each slice.

The Road Ahead

As you begin this journey into the world of real sourdough, I want you to remember that it's not about perfection. Baking real sourdough is an art as much as it is a science, and like any art, it takes time to master. You'll have loaves that don't rise, dough that feels too sticky, and maybe even the occasional burnt crust—but that's okay. The process of learning and improving is part of the joy. Every loaf you bake brings you one step closer to a healthier, stronger, and more vibrant you.

In the chapters ahead, you'll not only learn how to bake sourdough but also understand why real sourdough is essential for a balanced, healthy lifestyle. By the end of this book, I hope you'll feel confident in the kitchen, inspired to create your own healing sourdough breads, and empowered to take charge of your health in the most delicious way possible.

Let's get started on this journey together, and remember: real sourdough heals.

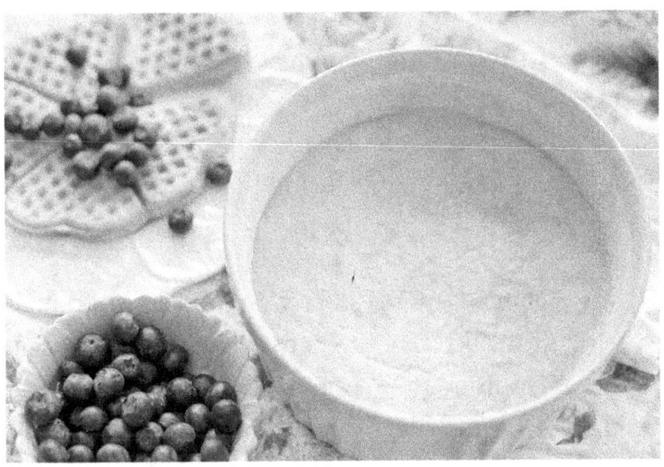

Chapter 1: What is Real Sourdough?

Sourdough bread has been a foundational part of the human diet for millennia. Yet, in recent decades, the sourdough we see on most grocery store shelves barely resembles what our ancestors ate. What was once a nourishing, wholesome food has often been reduced to little more than a convenient, processed filler. But real sourdough—simple, natural, and traditionally prepared—is still within our reach, and it holds the key to better health, greater vitality, and a deeper connection to our food.

In this chapter, we'll explore what makes sourdough "real," the differences between traditional and modern sourdough , and the ingredients that transform simple dough into a source of healing for the body and mind.

The Essence of Real Sourdough

So, what exactly is real sourdough ? At its core, real Sourdough is made from just a few simple, natural ingredients: flour, water, salt, and a leavening agent, such as wild yeast or a sourdough starter. These ingredients are then carefully combined and left to ferment, often over many hours or even days, allowing the sourdough to develop its complex flavor and texture. Unlike modern, mass-produced Sourdough , which is churned out in a matter of hours, real sourdough is the product of time, patience, and care.

But real sourdough is more than just the sum of its ingredients. It's about the process. Traditional sourdough -making methods, especially long fermentation, unlock the nutritional potential of the grains used in the dough. The long rise time allows the yeast and bacteria in the dough to break down the gluten and make the sourdough more digestible. This process also produces beneficial bacteria, or probiotics, that promote gut health and support the body's natural healing processes.

Real sourdough is not just about avoiding additives and chemicals; it's about creating food that nourishes, heals, and sustains us. It's about returning to simplicity and rejecting the convenience-driven shortcuts of modern food production.

How Real Sourdough Differs from Modern Sourdough

The sourdough you see in most supermarkets is, in reality, far removed from what real Sourdough should be. The primary goal of industrial Sourdough -making is speed and efficiency, not nutrition or flavor. Mass-produced sourdough is often made with refined, bleached flour that has been stripped of its natural nutrients, leaving behind little more than empty calories. Commercial bakers use fast-acting yeast to speed up the rise time, skipping the long fermentation process that makes sourdough easier to digest and more nutritious.

Modern sourdough is also loaded with preservatives, additives, and artificial flavors. These ingredients are added to extend the shelf life, improve the texture, and make the sourdough look and taste appealing even though it's far from its natural state. Sugar, high-fructose corn syrup, and other sweeteners are often included to mask the blandness of the processed flour, creating a product that's highly palatable but ultimately detrimental to our health.

Unlike real sourdough , which supports digestive health and provides sustained energy, modern Sourdough can lead to a host of health problems. The refined flour and added sugars cause blood sugar spikes, which can lead to energy crashes, weight gain, and an increased risk of conditions like type 2 diabetes and heart disease. For many people, modern sourdough can also cause digestive discomfort, such as bloating and indigestion, due to the high gluten content and lack of fermentation.

Real sourdough , on the other hand, nourishes the body with its natural, whole ingredients. It provides a rich source of fiber, vitamins, and minerals, and the fermentation process enhances its nutritional value. When you choose real Sourdough , you're not just eating to fill your stomach—you're eating to heal, energize, and thrive.

A Short History of Sourdough Baking

To truly understand real sourdough , it's important to appreciate its long history. Sourdough has been a staple food for thousands of years, dating back to ancient civilizations. The earliest Sourdough was likely made over 12,000 years ago by crushing wild grains and mixing them with water to form a paste that was then cooked over a fire. These early flatSourdough s were simple and nourishing, providing essential sustenance for ancient peoples.

The invention of leavened Sourdough , which rises and becomes light and airy, is believed to have occurred in ancient Egypt around 3,000 BC. Egyptian bakers discovered that wild yeast from the air could ferment the dough, causing it to rise. This discovery transformed sourdough-making, allowing for the creation of the soft, fluffy loaves that we still enjoy today.

Throughout history, sourdough has been a symbol of sustenance and community. In many cultures, Sourdough is considered sacred and plays a central role in religious rituals and celebrations. The phrase "breaking sourdough " is synonymous with sharing a meal and fostering connection.

Traditional sourdough -making methods were passed down from generation to generation, each culture developing its own unique techniques and recipes. For centuries, Sourdough was made by hand, often using sourdough starters or other natural leavening agents that promoted slow fermentation and enhanced the flavor and nutrition of the sourdough.

It wasn't until the Industrial Revolution in the 19th century that the process of making sourdough began to change dramatically. The invention of the mechanical sourdough mixer, commercial yeast, and the mass production of white flour allowed bakers to produce Sourdough on a much larger scale. While these innovations made sourdough more widely available and affordable, they also stripped away much of the nutritional value and artistry that had defined sourdough for thousands of years.

Ingredients That Heal

One of the key differences between real sourdough and its modern counterpart lies in the ingredients. The simplicity of real sourdough's ingredients is what makes it so powerful, and each one plays a crucial role in promoting health and healing.

Flour: Real sourdough begins with high-quality flour, ideally from whole grains. Whole grains contain all three parts of the grain—the bran, germ, and endosperm—which means they retain their fiber, vitamins, minerals, and antioxidants. In contrast, refined white flour is made by removing the bran and germ, which strips away most of the grain's nutritional value. Whole grain flour, especially when made from ancient grains like spelt, einkorn, and emmer, provides a rich source of nutrients that support digestion, heart health, and overall wellness.

Water: While it may seem like a simple ingredient, water is critical to the sourdough -making process. The type and quality of water you use can influence the texture and flavor of your sourdough. In real sourdough, water helps activate the yeast or sourdough starter, allowing the dough to ferment and rise naturally. It also hydrates the flour, helping to develop the gluten and create the sourdough's structure.

Salt: Salt not only enhances the flavor of the Sourdough but also plays a role in controlling the fermentation process. In real sourdough, unrefined sea salt or mineral-rich salts are often used to provide essential electrolytes and trace minerals that support health. Commercial sourdough, on the other hand, often contains excessive amounts of sodium and artificial additives, contributing to health problems like high blood pressure.

Yeast or Sourdough Starter: The leavening agent is what makes Sourdough rise, and in real sourdough, this is typically wild yeast from a sourdough starter or natural yeast found in the environment. Sourdough starters are a living culture of wild yeast and beneficial bacteria, and they play a critical role in real sourdough's health benefits. During the fermentation process, the wild yeast breaks down gluten, making the sourdough easier to digest. The beneficial bacteria also produce lactic acid, which lowers the Sourdough 's glycemic index and makes it more gut-friendly. Sourdough fermentation also increases the bioavailability of nutrients in the Sourdough , making it more nourishing for the body.

Together, these simple ingredients create a food that not only tastes delicious but also promotes healing from the inside out. By choosing whole, unprocessed ingredients and allowing the sourdough to ferment naturally, you're creating something that truly nourishes the body and supports overall wellness.

The Revival of Real Sourdough

Fortunately, we are in the midst of a real sourdough revival. Around the world, people are rediscovering the art of traditional sourdough -making, and small-scale bakers are returning to time-honored techniques. This movement is about more than just nostalgia—it's a response to the growing awareness that modern food systems are failing us. People are waking up to the fact that what we eat has a profound impact on our health, and they're seeking out real, nourishing foods to replace the processed, unhealthy options that dominate our diets.

The real sourdough movement is also about sustainability. Large-scale Sourdough production is incredibly resource-intensive and often relies on monoculture farming, which depletes the soil and contributes to environmental degradation. In contrast, real sourdough is often made with locally grown, organic grains, and the slow fermentation process requires far less energy than the rapid, industrial methods used in commercial sourdough production.

By choosing real sourdough , you're not only supporting your health—you're also supporting a more sustainable and ethical food system. You're voting with your fork, and each loaf of real Sourdough you bake or buy is a small step toward a healthier, more sustainable future.

The Power of Sourdough to Transform Health

Sourdough has the power to heal, but not just in a metaphorical sense. Real Sourdough , made with care and whole ingredients, can have a profound impact on your physical health.

One of the key benefits of real sourdough is its ability to support digestive health. The fermentation process involved in making sourdough or other naturally leavened sourdoughs creates probiotics, which are beneficial bacteria that help maintain a healthy gut microbiome. A balanced microbiome is essential for proper digestion, immune function, and even mental health. Studies have shown that a healthy gut can reduce inflammation, improve mood, and protect against diseases like irritable bowel syndrome and autoimmune disorders.

Real sourdough can also help balance blood sugar levels. Unlike highly processed sourdough made from refined white flour, real sourdough made from whole grains has a low glycemic index, which means it releases sugar slowly into the bloodstream. This helps prevent the sharp spikes and crashes in blood sugar that are common with modern Sourdough , reducing the risk of insulin resistance, type 2 diabetes, and weight gain.

In addition, real sourdough provides sustained energy. The complex carbohydrates found in whole grains are broken down slowly by the body, providing a steady source of fuel throughout the day. This makes real sourdough an ideal choice for anyone looking to improve their physical performance, whether in sports, work, or daily life.

Finally, real sourdough is rich in vitamins and minerals that support overall health. Whole grains are a natural source of B vitamins, which are essential for energy production, brain function, and the formation of red blood cells. They also contain important minerals like iron, magnesium, and zinc, which support immune function, bone health, and muscle strength.

Chapter 2: The Science Behind Real Sourdough

We often think of sourdough as a simple food—flour, water, salt, and yeast mixed together to create something we enjoy with our meals. But behind every loaf of real sourdough is a complex and fascinating scientific process. When we use whole grains and natural fermentation methods, the results go far beyond a satisfying flavor and texture. The science behind real sourdough explains why it is not just food for the body, but also medicine for our gut, our immune system, and even our mental health.

In this chapter, we'll dive into the science behind real sourdough, focusing on how ancient grains and traditional sourdough -making techniques impact our bodies on a deeper level. We'll explore the gut-brain connection, the nutritional value of whole grains, and the surprising ways real sourdough can improve both physical and mental wellness.

The Gut and Grain Connection

The digestive system is often referred to as the body's second brain, and for good reason. Our gut is home to trillions of bacteria, known as the gut microbiome, which play a critical role in our overall health. This microbiome helps with digestion, supports the immune system, and even influences our mood and cognitive function.

Real sourdough , particularly when made using sourdough fermentation, can have a powerful positive impact on the gut microbiome. The long fermentation process involved in making sourdough creates an ideal environment for beneficial bacteria to thrive. These bacteria, known as probiotics, help populate the gut with friendly microbes that aid in digestion and support a healthy immune response.

One of the key benefits of sourdough fermentation is its ability to break down gluten and make the sourdough easier to digest. Gluten, a protein found in wheat and other grains, is often blamed for causing digestive problems such as bloating, gas, and discomfort, particularly in people with gluten sensitivities or intolerances. However, sourdough fermentation breaks down much of the gluten before the sourdough is baked, making it more digestible for many people who otherwise struggle with gluten-rich foods.

In addition to aiding in digestion, the probiotics produced during fermentation help maintain the balance of bacteria in the gut, promoting a healthy gut microbiome. A balanced microbiome is essential for preventing a wide range of health issues, including digestive disorders, inflammation, and even mood disorders like anxiety and depression. This gut-brain connection is one of the reasons why many people report feeling better not only physically but also mentally after switching to real sourdough.

The Role of Fiber in Gut Health

Another significant way real sourdough supports gut health is through its high fiber content. Unlike processed Sourdough made from refined flour, real Sourdough made with whole grains retains all of the grain's natural fiber. This fiber plays a crucial role in digestive health, helping to move food through the digestive system and promoting regular bowel movements.

But fiber does more than just keep your digestion regular. It also acts as a prebiotic, providing food for the good bacteria in your gut. By feeding these beneficial bacteria, fiber helps them thrive, which in turn supports a healthy, balanced gut microbiome. A diet rich in prebiotic fiber from whole grains can help reduce inflammation in the gut, lower the risk of colon cancer, and improve overall digestion.

Studies have shown that consuming whole grains like those found in real Sourdough can increase the diversity of the gut microbiome, which is linked to better overall health. A diverse microbiome is more resilient and better able to protect against harmful bacteria, viruses, and other pathogens. This means that by eating real sourdough, you're not just improving your digestion—you're also boosting your immune system and reducing your risk of chronic diseases.

Nutritional Benefits of Ancient Grains

While modern sourdough is typically made from refined white flour, which has been stripped of its nutrients, real sourdough often uses whole grains or ancient grains like spelt, einkorn, and emmer. These grains are nutritionally dense and offer a wide range of health benefits that are absent in refined grains.

Spelt: Spelt is an ancient grain that has been cultivated for thousands of years. It is rich in fiber, protein, and essential minerals like magnesium, iron, and zinc. The high fiber content in spelt helps regulate blood sugar levels and supports healthy digestion, while its protein content makes it a great choice for those looking to maintain muscle mass and strength. Spelt also contains a variety of B vitamins, which are important for energy production and brain health.

Einkorn: Einkorn is considered one of the oldest cultivated grains, and it has remained largely unchanged for thousands of years. It is higher in protein and lower in gluten than modern wheat, making it easier to digest for many people. Einkorn is also rich in antioxidants, which help protect the body from oxidative stress and reduce the risk of chronic diseases like heart disease and cancer.

Emmer: Emmer, also known as farro, is another ancient grain that offers a rich source of fiber, protein, and essential nutrients like magnesium, phosphorus, and iron. Like other ancient grains, emmer is more nutrient-dense than modern wheat and has a lower glycemic index, meaning it helps stabilize blood sugar levels and provides sustained energy.

These ancient grains are less processed and closer to their original form, which means they retain more of their natural nutrients. When used in real Sourdough , they provide a wealth of vitamins, minerals, and antioxidants that support overall health.

Sourdough and Mental Wellness

While we typically think of food's impact on our physical health, real Sourdough can also play a significant role in supporting mental wellness. The gut-brain connection, which refers to the way the gut and brain communicate with each other, is a major factor in how our diet affects our mental health. The gut produces about 90% of the body's serotonin, a neurotransmitter that plays a key role in regulating mood, sleep, and appetite. When our gut health is compromised, our mental health can suffer as well.

Real Sourdough , particularly when made with whole grains and fermented naturally, can help support the production of serotonin and other neurotransmitters. The beneficial bacteria produced during fermentation help maintain a healthy gut, which in turn supports healthy brain function. This is why many people report feeling happier, calmer, and more focused after switching to real Sourdough made with natural ingredients.

In addition to its impact on serotonin production, real Sourdough also provides a steady source of complex carbohydrates, which are essential for brain function. The brain relies on glucose, a simple sugar, for energy, and the slow digestion of complex carbohydrates in real Sourdough ensures a steady supply of glucose to the brain. This helps prevent the mood swings and energy crashes that are often associated with eating refined, high-sugar foods like processed Sourdough .

Real Sourdough also contains important nutrients like B vitamins, magnesium, and zinc, which are essential for brain health and function. B vitamins, in particular, play a key role in the production of neurotransmitters, while magnesium helps regulate stress and improve sleep. Zinc is involved in the production of brain chemicals that affect mood and cognition.

By supporting gut health, providing essential nutrients, and promoting a steady supply of energy to the brain, real Sourdough can have a profound impact on mental wellness. It's not just food for the body—it's food for the mind as well.

How Real Sourdough Boosts the Immune System

In today's world, maintaining a strong immune system is more important than ever. Real Sourdough can help support immune function in several ways, making it a valuable addition to a health-focused diet.

The fermentation process used in making real Sourdough produces lactic acid, which has been shown to have antimicrobial properties. This means that real Sourdough can help protect the body from harmful bacteria and viruses, reducing the risk of infections and illnesses. In addition, the probiotics produced during fermentation support the health of the gut microbiome, which plays a critical role in immune function.

A healthy gut is essential for a strong immune system. The gut is home to about 70% of the body's immune cells, and the balance of bacteria in the gut can influence how well the immune system functions. When the gut microbiome is healthy and balanced, the immune system is better able to respond to threats and protect the body from illness.

In addition to supporting gut health, real Sourdough made with whole grains provides essential nutrients like zinc, selenium, and iron, which are critical for immune function. Zinc helps regulate the immune response and supports the body's ability to fight off infections. Selenium is a powerful antioxidant that helps protect immune cells from damage, while iron is essential for the production of immune cells.

By supporting gut health, providing important nutrients, and offering antimicrobial benefits, real Sourdough can help strengthen the immune system and protect against illness.

Balancing Blood Sugar with Real Sourdough

One of the biggest health issues associated with modern Sourdough is its impact on blood sugar levels. Processed Sourdough made with refined white flour is quickly digested, causing a rapid spike in blood sugar levels. This spike is often followed by a sharp drop, leaving you feeling tired, hungry, and craving more sugar. Over time, these blood sugar fluctuations can lead to insulin resistance, weight gain, and an increased risk of type 2 diabetes.

Real Sourdough , on the other hand, is made with whole grains and fermented slowly, resulting in a lower glycemic index. The glycemic index (GI) measures how quickly a food raises blood sugar levels. Foods with a high GI, like white Sourdough , cause rapid spikes in blood sugar, while foods with a low GI, like real Sourdough , release sugar more slowly into the bloodstream.

The slow fermentation process used in making real Sourdough breaks down the starches in the flour, reducing the glycemic load of the Sourdough . This means that real Sourdough causes a slower, more controlled release of sugar into the bloodstream, helping to prevent blood sugar spikes and crashes.

Eating real Sourdough made from whole grains can help stabilize blood sugar levels, reduce cravings for sugary foods, and provide sustained energy throughout the day. This makes real Sourdough an excellent choice for people looking to manage their blood sugar levels and reduce their risk of developing insulin resistance or type 2 diabetes.

The Anti-Aging Properties of Real Sourdough

One of the most surprising benefits of real Sourdough is its ability to support healthy aging. While Sourdough is often thought of as a food to avoid for those concerned with weight gain or aging, real Sourdough made with whole grains and fermented naturally can actually have anti-aging properties.

Whole grains are rich in antioxidants, which help protect the body from oxidative stress and reduce inflammation. Oxidative stress is a major factor in the aging process, contributing to the development of chronic diseases like heart disease, cancer, and Alzheimer's disease. By providing a rich source of antioxidants, real Sourdough can help protect the body from the damaging effects of oxidative stress and support healthy aging.

In addition to its antioxidant content, real Sourdough also provides important nutrients like vitamin E, which is known for its anti-aging properties. Vitamin E helps protect the skin from damage caused by free radicals, reducing the appearance of wrinkles and promoting a more youthful complexion.

The fiber in real Sourdough also supports healthy aging by promoting heart health. Studies have shown that a diet rich in whole grains can reduce the risk of heart disease by lowering cholesterol levels, reducing inflammation, and improving blood pressure. By supporting heart health and reducing the risk of chronic diseases, real Sourdough can help you feel healthier and more youthful as you age.

Chapter 3: Sourdough as Medicine: Healing Your Body from Within

Sourdough bread is an ancient, time-honored staple of human diets, and while it's widely appreciated for its flavor and texture, what many don't realize is the profound impact it can have on health. As we continue to understand the importance of gut health, immunity, and balanced nutrition, sourdough's natural fermentation process emerges as a valuable tool in supporting overall well-being. We live in an age where chronic illnesses are on the rise, many of which are linked to poor diet, processed foods, and lifestyle choices. While modern medicine focuses on treating symptoms, there is growing evidence that prevention through proper nutrition is one of the most effective ways to maintain health and vitality. One of the simplest yet most profound ways to support your body's natural healing processes is by returning to real, unprocessed foods—starting with Sourdough . Real sourdough, when made with natural ingredients and fermented properly, can provide a range of health benefits that extend far beyond simple nourishment.

This chapter delves into how sourdough can serve as a form of "medicine," aiding digestion, enhancing immunity, boosting energy, and even playing a role in weight management. We'll explore how real sourdough contributes to better health in multiple ways, from boosting the immune system to supporting heart health and maintaining stable blood sugar levels. We'll also look at how the nutrients found in whole grains and fermented sourdough breads help you age gracefully and provide long-lasting energy for an active life.

Boost Your Immune System

The immune system is your body's first line of defense against infections, viruses, and other pathogens. A strong immune system is essential for preventing illness and staying healthy, and real Sourdough can play an important role in supporting immune function.

One of the most significant ways real sourdough helps boost the immune system is through its impact on the gut microbiome. As we discussed in the previous chapter, the gut is home to trillions of bacteria, many of which are crucial for maintaining immune health. Approximately 70% of the body's immune cells are found in the gut, and these cells rely on a balanced microbiome to function properly.

When you eat real sourdough made with fermented dough, such as sourdough, you're introducing beneficial bacteria (probiotics) into your gut. These probiotics help maintain the balance of good bacteria in your digestive system, which in turn supports the immune system. A healthy gut microbiome ensures that your immune system is better equipped to respond to infections, fight off harmful pathogens, and prevent inflammation.

In addition to supporting gut health, real Sourdough made with whole grains provides essential nutrients that are critical for immune function. Whole grains are rich in vitamins and minerals, particularly zinc, selenium, and B vitamins, which play key roles in immune regulation.

Zinc: This mineral is essential for immune health, as it helps regulate the immune response and supports the function of immune cells. Zinc deficiency has been linked to a weakened immune system and increased susceptibility to infections. Real Sourdough made from whole grains like spelt and einkorn is a good source of zinc, providing a natural way to support immune health.

Selenium: Selenium is a powerful antioxidant that protects immune cells from oxidative damage. It also plays a crucial role in the production of cytokines, which are proteins that help regulate the immune response. Whole grain Sourdough is a good source of selenium, helping to keep the immune system strong and resilient.

B Vitamins: B vitamins, particularly B6, B9 (folate), and B12, are essential for the production of white blood cells, which are the body's primary defense against infections. Real Sourdough made from whole grains is rich in B vitamins, helping to support the production of these immune-boosting cells.

By regularly incorporating real Sourdough into your diet, you're not only nourishing your body with essential nutrients but also giving your immune system the tools it needs to protect you from illness and keep you healthy.

Age Gracefully with Real Sourdough

Aging is a natural process, but how we age—whether gracefully or with chronic illness and frailty—depends largely on our lifestyle choices, particularly our diet. Real Sourdough , made with whole grains and fermented naturally, offers a wealth of nutrients and health benefits that can help you age gracefully, maintain your strength, and feel youthful well into your later years.

One of the key factors in healthy aging is reducing inflammation in the body. Chronic inflammation has been linked to a variety of age-related diseases, including heart disease, Alzheimer's disease, and arthritis. Fortunately, the antioxidants and anti-inflammatory compounds found in whole grains can help reduce inflammation and protect the body from the damaging effects of oxidative stress.

Antioxidants: Whole grains used in real sourdough are rich in antioxidants, including vitamin E and selenium, which help neutralize free radicals—unstable molecules that cause cellular damage and contribute to aging. By consuming real Sourdough , you're giving your body the tools it needs to fight oxidative stress and protect against age-related diseases.

Fiber: Another important component of whole grains is fiber, which supports heart health by helping to lower cholesterol levels and regulate blood sugar. A diet high in fiber has been shown to reduce the risk of heart disease, which is one of the leading causes of death in older adults. In addition, fiber promotes healthy digestion, which becomes increasingly important as we age.

Magnesium: Real sourdough made from ancient grains like spelt and einkorn is a good source of magnesium, a mineral that is essential for muscle and nerve function. Magnesium also helps regulate blood pressure and supports bone health, making it an important nutrient for maintaining strength and mobility as you age.

By choosing real sourdough over processed, nutrient-poor options, you can help your body age more gracefully. The nutrients found in real Sourdough support heart health, brain function, and muscle strength, allowing you to stay active and vibrant as you grow older.

Balancing Blood Sugar Naturally

One of the most pressing health concerns in today's society is the rise of type 2 diabetes and metabolic syndrome, both of which are linked to poor dietary choices. The overconsumption of processed foods, particularly those made with refined carbohydrates and added sugars, has contributed to a dramatic increase in blood sugar imbalances and insulin resistance.

Processed sourdough, made with refined white flour, is one of the worst offenders when it comes to spiking blood sugar levels. Refined flour is quickly digested and absorbed into the bloodstream, causing a rapid rise in blood sugar. This is often followed by a crash, leaving you feeling tired, hungry, and craving more carbohydrates. Over time, these blood sugar spikes and crashes can lead to insulin resistance, weight gain, and an increased risk of developing type 2 diabetes.

Real sourdough , on the other hand, is made with whole grains and fermented slowly, which helps regulate blood sugar levels and reduce the risk of insulin resistance. The key to real Sourdough 's blood sugar-balancing properties lies in both its ingredients and its preparation method.

Whole Grains: Unlike refined flour, whole grains retain their fiber, which slows down the digestion and absorption of carbohydrates. This means that real Sourdough made with whole grains has a lower glycemic index (GI), which causes a slower, more gradual rise in blood sugar levels. This helps prevent the spikes and crashes associated with refined carbohydrates, providing steady energy throughout the day.

Fermentation: The fermentation process used in making sourdough and other real sourdoughs further reduces the glycemic load of the sourdough. During fermentation, the natural yeast and bacteria break down some of the starches in the flour, making the Sourdough easier to digest and less likely to cause blood sugar spikes. Fermentation also increases the bioavailability of nutrients in the sourdough, making it more nourishing for the body.

Eating real sourdough as part of a balanced diet can help stabilize blood sugar levels, reduce cravings for sugary foods, and support healthy weight management. For people at risk of developing diabetes or those who are already managing the condition, real sourdough is a much healthier alternative to the processed Sourdough s commonly found in stores.

Support for Heart Health

Heart disease remains one of the leading causes of death worldwide, but diet plays a crucial role in preventing and managing cardiovascular issues. One of the key components of a heart-healthy diet is whole grains, and real Sourdough made with these grains provides a wealth of nutrients that support heart health and reduce the risk of cardiovascular disease.

Fiber: Whole grains are an excellent source of dietary fiber, which has been shown to reduce cholesterol levels and improve heart health. Soluble fiber, in particular, helps lower LDL cholesterol (the "bad" cholesterol) by binding to cholesterol particles and removing them from the body. By incorporating real Sourdough into your diet, you can help lower your risk of heart disease and improve overall cardiovascular function.

Healthy Fats: Real sourdough can also be enhanced with heart-healthy ingredients like seeds, nuts, and olive oil. These ingredients provide unsaturated fats, which help reduce inflammation and lower the risk of heart disease. Seeds like flaxseeds and chia seeds are rich in omega-3 fatty acids, which have been shown to reduce blood pressure and prevent the buildup of plaque in the arteries.

Magnesium and Potassium: Real sourdough made with whole grains is a good source of magnesium and potassium, two minerals that are essential for maintaining healthy blood pressure. Magnesium helps relax blood vessels and improve circulation, while potassium helps balance sodium levels and prevent hypertension.

By choosing real sourdough over processed, refined Slsourdoughs, you're supporting your heart health with cach bite. The fiber, healthy fats, and essential minerals found in real Sourdough work together to reduce the risk of heart disease and promote cardiovascular wellness.

Long-Lasting Energy for Active Lifestyles

Whether you're an athlete, a busy professional, or someone with an active lifestyle, you need a steady source of energy to fuel your day. Real sourdough, made with whole grains and fermented slowly, provides long-lasting energy that supports physical performance and mental clarity.

The complex carbohydrates found in whole grains are broken down slowly by the body, providing a steady release of glucose into the bloodstream. This is in contrast to the rapid digestion of refined carbohydrates, which cause blood sugar spikes and crashes. By providing a sustained source of energy, real Sourdough helps you avoid the mid-afternoon energy slump and keeps you feeling focused and alert throughout the day.

In addition to its energy-sustaining properties, real Sourdough is rich in nutrients that support physical performance, including protein, B vitamins, and iron.

Protein: Real sourdough made with ancient grains like spelt and einkorn contains more protein than modern wheat, making it an excellent choice for those looking to maintain muscle mass and strength. Protein is essential for muscle repair and recovery, especially after exercise, and real Sourdough provides a natural, plant-based source of this important nutrient.

B Vitamins: B vitamins, particularly B1 (thiamine) and B3 (niacin), are essential for energy production.

These vitamins help convert carbohydrates into glucose, which the body uses for energy. Real Sourdough made with whole grains is a good source of B vitamins, helping to support your energy needs throughout the day.

Iron: Iron is critical for transporting oxygen to the muscles and tissues, which is especially important for athletes and those with active lifestyles. Real Sourdough made from whole grains provides a plant-based source of iron, helping to prevent fatigue and improve endurance.

Whether you're fueling up for a workout or powering through a busy day, real Sourdough provides the energy and nutrients your body needs to perform at its best.

Real Sourdough and Weight Management

One of the most persistent myths about sourdough is that it contributes to weight gain. While processed Sourdough made with refined flour and added sugars can certainly lead to weight gain, real Sourdough made with whole grains and natural ingredients can actually support healthy weight management.

The key to real sourdough's weight management benefits lies in its high fiber content and its ability to promote satiety. The fiber found in whole grains helps slow digestion, keeping you feeling fuller for longer. This reduces the likelihood of overeating or snacking on unhealthy foods between meals. In addition, the slow release of energy from real sourdough helps prevent the blood sugar spikes and crashes that often lead to cravings for sugary or high-calorie foods.

By choosing real sourdough made with whole grains, you can support your weight management goals without sacrificing flavor or satisfaction. Real Sourdough provides the nutrients and energy your body needs while helping you maintain a healthy weight.

Chapter 4: The Art of Baking Real Sourdough

There's something deeply satisfying about making your own sourdough. The process of mixing, kneading, and baking transforms simple ingredients into something nourishing and delicious. But when you make real sourdough, it's about more than just the taste. You're reconnecting with tradition, with nature, and with the food you eat. Real Sourdough , with its natural fermentation and whole grains, is a celebration of simplicity and time-honored techniques that have been passed down through generations.

In this chapter, we'll dive into the art of baking real sourdough, covering everything from selecting ingredients to mastering basic techniques. Whether you're a beginner baker or someone who's already comfortable in the kitchen, you'll find practical advice and detailed steps to guide you through the process of making your first loaf. Along the way, we'll also explore some of the challenges you might encounter and how to overcome them.

Getting Started with the Basics

Baking real Sourdough doesn't require fancy equipment or advanced skills, but it does require patience and attention to detail. Before you begin, it's important to understand the basic elements of real sourdough: flour, water, salt, and leavening (usually yeast or a sourdough starter). These four ingredients come together to form the foundation of real sourdough, and mastering them is the key to a great loaf.

1. Flour: Choosing the Right Grain

The type of flour you use will have a major impact on the texture, flavor, and nutrition of your dourdough. For real Sourdough , whole grain flours are the best choice because they retain all parts of the grain—the bran, germ, and endosperm—which means they're packed with fiber, vitamins, and minerals. When shopping for flour, look for options that are organic and minimally processed.

Wheat Flour: Whole wheat flour is a versatile option and can be used for most types of sourdough. It has a rich, nutty flavor and provides excellent structure for the dough.

Spelt Flour: Spelt is an ancient grain that's higher in protein and easier to digest than modern wheat. It has a slightly sweet, nutty flavor and makes a light, airy loaf.

Rye Flour: Rye flour is denser and lower in gluten than wheat, making it ideal for hearty, rustic sourdoughs. It's also rich in fiber and nutrients that support gut health.

Einkorn and Emmer: These ancient grains are known for their rich flavor and high nutritional value. They have a lower gluten content, making them easier to digest, but they require a bit more attention when baking due to their unique texture.

You can also experiment with mixing different flours to create your own signature blend. For example, combining whole wheat with spelt or rye can add depth of flavor and improve the texture of your sourdough.

2. Water: The Key to Hydration

Water may seem like a simple ingredient, but the amount you use can greatly affect the outcome of your sourdough. The ratio of water to flour, known as the dough's hydration, will determine how soft or firm your sourdough will be. A higher hydration level will result in a more open crumb (the holes inside the Sourdough), while a lower hydration will produce a denser loaf.

For most sourdough recipes, you'll want to use filtered or bottled water to avoid any unwanted minerals or chemicals that could affect the yeast's fermentation. Room temperature water is typically best for mixing, though some recipes may call for warm water to help activate the yeast.

3. Salt: Enhancing Flavor and Structure

Salt isn't just for seasoning—it also plays a vital role in controlling the fermentation process and strengthening the dough's structure. Without salt, Sourdough can taste flat and may rise too quickly, resulting in an uneven crumb. When using salt in sourdough-making, opt for natural sea salt or Himalayan salt, which contains trace minerals that add depth of flavor.

The amount of salt you use can vary depending on your taste preferences, but a general guideline is to use about 1.5 to 2% of the flour's weight in salt. For example, if your recipe calls for 500 grams of flour, you'll want to use about 7.5 to 10 grams of salt.

4. Leavening: Yeast or Sourdough Starter

Leavening is what causes your sourdough to rise, and there are two main methods for doing this: using commercial yeast or a sourdough starter.

Commercial Yeast: This is the most common type of leavening used in sourdough baking. It's fast-acting and reliable, which makes it ideal for beginners. Yeast comes in two main forms: active dry yeast (which needs to be dissolved in water before use) and instant yeast (which can be mixed directly into the dough).

Sourdough Starter: A sourdough starter is a natural leavening agent made from wild yeast and bacteria that naturally occur in flour and the environment. Using a starter adds a depth of flavor and improves the sourdough's digestibility by breaking down gluten during the fermentation process. While using a sourdough starter takes more time and care, the results are worth it for both flavor and health benefits.

Essential Tools for Real Sourdough Baking

To get started with baking real sourdough, you don't need a lot of specialized equipment. However, there are a few key tools that will make the process easier and help you achieve better results.

Mixing Bowls: You'll need a large mixing bowl for combining the ingredients and letting the dough rise. Stainless steel or glass bowls work best.

Digital Scale: Measuring your ingredients by weight rather than volume is more accurate and will lead to better results. A digital scale is essential for measuring flour, water, and other ingredients.

Dough Scraper: This handy tool helps you mix and knead the dough without sticking to your hands. It's also useful for shaping the dough and scraping it off your work surface.

Bench Knife: A bench knife, or bench scraper, is useful for dividing dough and handling sticky doughs.

Proofing Basket (Banneton): A proofing basket helps the dough hold its shape as it rises. It also leaves beautiful patterns on the surface of the Sourdough .

Dutch Oven: Many bakers prefer baking sourdough in a Dutch oven because it creates a steamy environment that helps the Sourdough develop a crisp crust. If you don't have a Dutch oven, you can also use a baking stone with a steam tray in the oven.

Lame or Sharp Knife: A lame is a tool used to score the top of the dough before baking, which helps control how the sourdough expands in the oven. If you don't have a lame, a very sharp knife will work as well.

Step-by-Step Guide to Making Your First Loaf

Now that you've gathered your ingredients and tools, it's time to bake your first loaf of real sourdough. For this guide, we'll focus on a basic whole wheat sourdough loaf, but the principles can be applied to other types of sourdough as well.

Step 1: Mix the Dough

Start by weighing out your ingredients:

- 500 grams of whole wheat flour
- 350 grams of water
- 100 grams of sourdough starter (fed and active)
- 10 grams of salt

In a large mixing bowl, combine the flour and water. Mix until there are no dry patches of flour left, then cover the bowl with a damp towel and let it sit for 30 minutes. This rest period, called **autolyse**, allows the flour to fully hydrate and helps develop the dough's gluten.

After the autolyse, add the salt and sourdough starter to the dough. Using your hands, gently fold and stretch the dough to incorporate the ingredients. Continue folding the dough for about 5-10 minutes until it becomes smooth and elastic.

Step 2: Bulk Fermentation

Once your dough is mixed, it's time for the first rise, known as the **bulk fermentation**. Cover the bowl with a damp towel and let the dough rest at room temperature for 4-6 hours, depending on the temperature of your kitchen. During this time, the dough will rise and develop its flavor.

To help the dough rise evenly, perform **stretches and folds** every 30 minutes during the first 2 hours of bulk fermentation. To do this, grab one side of the dough, stretch it upward, and fold it over the rest of the dough. Turn the bowl a quarter turn and repeat on the other three sides. This helps build strength and structure in the dough without overworking it.

Step 3: Shaping the Dough

After the bulk fermentation, your dough should have risen and become airy. Turn the dough out onto a lightly floured surface and gently shape it into a round or oval shape, depending on the type of loaf you want. Use your hands to gently tuck the edges of the dough underneath, creating surface tension on the top of the loaf.

Once shaped, place the dough in a proofing basket or a bowl lined with a floured towel. Cover the dough and let it rest for 1-2 hours for the **final proof**, or refrigerate it overnight to develop even more flavor.

Step 4: Preheat the Oven

While your dough is finishing its final proof, preheat your oven to 475°F (245°C). If you're using a Dutch oven, place it in the oven to preheat as well. A hot Dutch oven helps create the steam needed for a crispy crust.

Step 5: Scoring the Dough

Before baking, you'll need to score the top of your dough to control how it expands in the oven. Turn the dough out of the proofing basket onto a piece of parchment paper. Using a lame or sharp knife, make a few deep cuts on the surface of the dough. Be bold with your scoring, as this will prevent the sourdough from bursting unevenly during baking.

Step 6: Bake the Sourdough

Carefully transfer the dough to the preheated Dutch oven. Cover the Dutch oven with its lid and bake for 20 minutes. After 20 minutes, remove the lid to allow the Sourdough to develop a golden crust. Continue baking for another 20-25 minutes until the Sourdough is deep brown and sounds hollow when tapped on the bottom.

If you're not using a Dutch oven, place your dough on a baking stone or baking sheet, and add a tray of hot water to the bottom of the oven to create steam.

Step 7: Let It Cool

Once your Sourdough is finished baking, remove it from the oven and transfer it to a cooling rack. As tempting as it may be, resist the urge to slice into the sourdough right away. Letting the sourdough cool for at least an hour allows the crumb to set and ensures a better texture.

Troubleshooting Common Issues

Sourdough baking is both an art and a science, and sometimes things don't go as planned. Here are a few common issues you might encounter and how to fix them:

Dense or Heavy Loaf: This can be caused by under-proofing the dough or not allowing enough fermentation time. Make sure your dough has risen properly during bulk fermentation and final proofing.

Flat or Spread-Out Loaf: If your dough spreads out rather than holding its shape, it may be over-proofed or too wet. Adjust your hydration level and proofing times as needed.

Pale Crust: A pale crust can result from baking at too low a temperature or not allowing enough steam in the oven. Ensure your oven is hot enough, and use a Dutch oven or steam tray to create a crisp, golden crust.

Fermentation and Sourdough Magic

The real magic of sourdough-making lies in fermentation. While commercial yeast works quickly, sourdough fermentation takes its time, allowing the wild yeast and bacteria in the starter to slowly break down the dough. This long, slow fermentation not only creates a more complex flavor but also enhances the sourdough's nutritional value.

Sourdough fermentation increases the bioavailability of nutrients in the Sourdough , making it easier for your body to absorb vitamins and minerals. It also helps reduce the gluten content, making sourdough easier to digest for many people who are sensitive to gluten.

If you're new to sourdough, creating and maintaining a starter may seem intimidating, but it's simpler than it sounds. All you need is flour, water, and time. With a little care, your starter will become the foundation of many delicious and nourishing loaves.

Chapter 5: The Power of Sourdough Bread

Sourdough bread has been a staple in traditional diets for centuries. It's made using a natural fermentation process that gives the Sourdough a unique flavor and texture, while also boosting its nutritional value. Unlike commercial sourdough, which relies on fast-acting yeast, sourdough uses wild yeast and beneficial bacteria that are present in the environment. This slow fermentation process breaks down gluten, enhances the bioavailability of nutrients, and makes sourdough easier to digest than conventional sourdough.

In this chapter, you'll find a variety of sourdough recipes, ranging from a basic loaf to more adventurous creations. Each recipe focuses on the use of whole grains, providing maximum flavor and health benefits. Let's dive into the magic of sourdough and start baking!

Recipe 1: Basic Whole Wheat Sourdough Bread

This is the perfect recipe for beginners who want to experience the benefits of sourdough while keeping things simple. With just a few ingredients and patience, you can create a loaf that's both nutritious and delicious.

Prep Time: 20 minutes (active)

Cook Time: 45 minutes

Total Time: 10-12 hours (including fermentation and proofing)

Servings: 1 loaf (about 10 slices)

Ingredients:

- 500 grams whole wheat flour
- 350 grams water (room temperature)
- 100 grams active sourdough starter (fed and bubbly)
- 10 grams sea salt

Instructions:

Mix the Dough: In a large mixing bowl, combine the whole wheat flour and water. Mix until there are no dry spots. Cover with a damp towel and let the mixture rest for 30 minutes (autolyse).

Add Starter and Salt: After the autolyse, add the sourdough starter and salt to the dough. Mix the ingredients together by folding the dough onto itself. Continue folding for about 5-10 minutes until the dough becomes smooth and elastic.

Bulk Fermentation: Cover the bowl with a damp towel and let the dough rise at room temperature for 4-6 hours, depending on the ambient temperature. Every 30 minutes for the first 2 hours, perform a series of stretch-and-folds (grab one side of the dough, stretch it up, and fold it over the center, repeating on all sides).

Shaping: After the dough has risen, transfer it to a lightly floured surface. Shape the dough into a round or oval loaf by gently pulling the edges toward the center to create tension on the surface. Place the shaped dough into a floured proofing basket (or a bowl lined with a floured towel).

Final Proof: Cover the dough and let it proof at room temperature for 1-2 hours, or refrigerate overnight for an even longer ferment, which enhances flavor.

Preheat the Oven: Preheat your oven to 475°F (245°C) with a Dutch oven inside.

Scoring and Baking: Once your dough is ready, carefully transfer it from the proofing basket onto a piece of parchment paper. Score the top of the dough with a sharp knife or lame. Place the dough into the preheated Dutch oven, cover with the lid, and bake for 20 minutes. Remove the lid and bake for an additional 25-30 minutes until the crust is deep golden brown.

Cooling: Remove the Sourdough from the oven and transfer it to a wire rack to cool completely before slicing.

Recipe 2: Sourdough Rye Bread

This dense, hearty rye loaf is rich in flavor and packed with nutrients. Rye flour contains less gluten than wheat, so it creates a tighter crumb with a chewy texture, making it perfect for sandwiches or toast.

Prep Time: 25 minutes (active)

Cook Time: 45 minutes

Total Time: 12-14 hours (including fermentation and proofing)

Servings: 1 loaf (about 10 slices)

Ingredients:

- 300 grams rye flour
- 200 grams whole wheat flour

- 375 grams water
- 100 grams active sourdough starter
- 12 grams sea salt
- 1 tablespoon caraway seeds (optional)

Instructions:

Mix the Dough: In a large bowl, combine the rye flour, whole wheat flour, and water. Mix until fully combined and cover with a damp towel. Let the dough rest for 30 minutes (autolyse).

Add Starter and Salt: After the autolyse, mix in the sourdough starter, salt, and caraway seeds (if using). Fold the dough onto itself until the ingredients are evenly incorporated. The dough will be sticky and dense, which is normal for rye Sourdough .

Bulk Fermentation: Cover the dough and let it ferment at room temperature for 4-6 hours. Every 30 minutes during the first 2 hours, perform a series of stretch-and-folds.

Shaping: Once the dough has doubled in size, shape it into a round or oval loaf. Place the shaped dough in a floured proofing basket, cover, and let it proof for another 1-2 hours or overnight in the refrigerator.

Preheat the Oven: Preheat your oven to 450°F (230°C) with a Dutch oven inside.

Scoring and Baking: Score the dough with a sharp knife or lame, then carefully transfer it to the Dutch oven. Cover and bake for 20 minutes. Remove the lid and bake for another 25 minutes until the crust is dark brown and firm.

Cooling: Let the loaf cool on a wire rack for at least an hour before slicing.

Recipe 3: Sourdough Spelt Bread with Seeds

Spelt is an ancient grain with a sweet, nutty flavor and high nutritional value. This recipe includes a mix of seeds for added texture and nutrients, making it a great option for a wholesome, hearty loaf.

Prep Time: 30 minutes (active)

Cook Time: 40 minutes

Total Time: 10-12 hours (including fermentation and proofing)

Servings: 1 loaf (about 12 slices)

Ingredients:

- 400 grams spelt flour
- 100 grams whole wheat flour
- 350 grams water
- 100 grams active sourdough starter
- 10 grams sea salt
- 50 grams sunflower seeds
- 25 grams flaxseeds
- 25 grams sesame seeds
- 1 tablespoon olive oil (optional)

Instructions:

Prepare the Seed Mix: In a small bowl, mix the sunflower seeds, flaxseeds, and sesame seeds. Set aside.

Mix the Dough: In a large bowl, combine the spelt flour, whole wheat flour, and water. Mix until well combined and let it rest for 30 minutes (autolyse).

Incorporate the Starter and Salt: After the autolyse, mix in the sourdough starter and salt. Fold the dough onto itself until smooth. If desired, add the olive oil to enhance the texture and flavor.

Add the Seeds: Gently fold the seed mixture into the dough until evenly distributed.

Bulk Fermentation: Cover the dough and let it rise at room temperature for 4-6 hours, performing stretch-and-folds every 30 minutes during the first 2 hours.

Shaping: Shape the dough into a loaf and place it into a proofing basket or bowl lined with a floured towel. Let it proof for 1-2 hours or overnight in the refrigerator.

Preheat the Oven: Preheat your oven to 450°F (230°C) with a Dutch oven inside.

Scoring and Baking: Score the dough, then transfer it to the Dutch oven. Bake with the lid on for 20 minutes. Remove the lid and bake for another 20-25 minutes until golden brown.

Cooling: Cool the Sourdough completely on a wire rack before slicing and serving.

Recipe 4: Sourdough Focaccia with Herbs

Focaccia is a flatSourdough that's perfect for dipping or serving with soups and salads. This sourdough version is airy, flavorful, and topped with herbs and olive oil for an added burst of flavor.

Prep Time: 20 minutes (active)

Cook Time: 25 minutes

Total Time: 8-10 hours (including fermentation and proofing)

Servings: 1 large focaccia (about 12 pieces)

Ingredients:

- 450 grams all-purpose flour or Sourdough flour
- 300 grams water
- 100 grams active sourdough starter
- 10 grams sea salt
- 4 tablespoons olive oil (plus more for drizzling)
- Fresh rosemary, thyme, and oregano (to taste)
- Flaky sea salt for sprinkling

Instructions:

Mix the Dough: In a large mixing bowl, combine the flour, water, sourdough starter, and sea salt. Mix until the ingredients come together into a sticky dough. Drizzle in 2 tablespoons of olive oil and mix until smooth.

Bulk Fermentation: Cover the dough with a damp towel and let it rise at room temperature for 6-8 hours, or until doubled in size. Perform 3-4 rounds of stretch-and-folds during the first 2 hours of fermentation.

Shape the Focaccia: Drizzle 2 tablespoons of olive oil into a baking tray or cast iron skillet. Gently transfer the dough into the tray and use your fingers to spread it out evenly, creating dimples on the surface. Let the dough rest for 1-2 hours.

Preheat the Oven: Preheat your oven to 450°F (230°C).

Add Toppings: Before baking, drizzle more olive oil over the dough and sprinkle with fresh herbs and flaky sea salt.

Bake: Bake for 20-25 minutes until golden brown and crispy on the edges.

Cooling: Allow the focaccia to cool slightly before cutting it into squares and serving.

Recipe 5: Multigrain Sourdough Bread

This multigrain sourdough loaf is packed with whole grains like oats, millet, and seeds, making it a nutrient-dense and flavorful Sourdough that's perfect for toast or sandwiches. It's a great way to add extra fiber, vitamins, and minerals to your diet.

Prep Time: 30 minutes (active)

Cook Time: 45 minutes

Total Time: 12-14 hours (including fermentation and proofing)

Servings: 1 loaf (about 12 slices)

Ingredients:

- 300 grams whole wheat flour
- 100 grams Sourdough flour
- 50 grams rolled oats
- 50 grams millet
- 375 grams water
- 100 grams active sourdough starter
- 10 grams sea salt
- 30 grams sunflower seeds
- 30 grams flaxseeds
- 2 tablespoons honey (optional)

Instructions:

Prepare the Grains: In a small bowl, soak the rolled oats, millet, and seeds in 100 grams of the water for 30 minutes.

Mix the Dough: In a large bowl, combine the whole wheat flour, Sourdough flour, remaining water, and honey (if using). Mix until combined, then cover and let the dough rest for 30 minutes (autolyse).

Incorporate the Starter and Salt: After the autolyse, add the sourdough starter and sea salt to the dough. Gently fold and mix until smooth.

Add the Soaked Grains: Drain any excess water from the soaked grains and seeds, then fold them into the dough until evenly distributed.

Bulk Fermentation: Cover the dough and let it rise at room temperature for 4-6 hours. Perform a series of stretch-and-folds every 30 minutes during the first 2 hours to strengthen the dough.

Shaping: Shape the dough into a round or oval loaf and place it into a proofing basket or bowl lined with a floured towel. Cover and let it proof at room temperature for 1-2 hours, or refrigerate overnight.

Preheat the Oven: Preheat the oven to 475°F (245°C) with a Dutch oven inside.

Scoring and Baking: Score the dough with a lame or sharp knife and carefully transfer it to the preheated Dutch oven. Bake with the lid on for 20 minutes, then remove the lid and bake for another 25 minutes until golden brown.

Cooling: Transfer the loaf to a wire rack and let it cool completely before slicing.

Recipe 6: Sourdough Cinnamon Raisin Bread

This slightly sweet sourdough bread is perfect for breakfast or a mid-afternoon snack. The combination of cinnamon and raisins gives it a warm, comforting flavor, while the sourdough starter adds complexity and depth.

Prep Time: 25 minutes (active)

Cook Time: 45 minutes

Total Time: 10-12 hours (including fermentation and proofing)

Servings: 1 loaf (about 10 slices)

Ingredients:

- 400 grams Sourdough flour
- 100 grams whole wheat flour
- 350 grams water
- 100 grams active sourdough starter
- 10 grams sea salt
- 2 tablespoons ground cinnamon
- 150 grams raisins

- 2 tablespoons honey or maple syrup (optional)
- 1 tablespoon butter (for greasing)

Instructions:

Soak the Raisins: In a small bowl, soak the raisins in warm water for 30 minutes, then drain and set aside.

Mix the Dough: In a large mixing bowl, combine the Sourdough flour, whole wheat flour, and water. Mix until combined and let the dough rest for 30 minutes.

Add Starter and Salt: After the autolyse, add the sourdough starter, sea salt, cinnamon, and honey (if using). Mix the dough until everything is evenly incorporated.

Add the Raisins: Gently fold the soaked raisins into the dough until evenly distributed.

Bulk Fermentation: Cover the dough and let it rise for 4-6 hours at room temperature. Perform stretch-and-folds every 30 minutes for the first 2 hours.

Shaping: Shape the dough into a round loaf and place it in a greased proofing basket or bowl lined with a floured towel. Let the dough proof at room temperature for 1-2 hours, or refrigerate overnight.

Preheat the Oven: Preheat your oven to 450°F (230°C) with a Dutch oven inside.

Scoring and Baking: Score the dough and carefully transfer it to the Dutch oven. Bake with the lid on for 20 minutes, then remove the lid and bake for another 20-25 minutes until the Sourdough is golden brown and fragrant.

Cooling: Allow the loaf to cool completely on a wire rack before slicing and enjoying.

Recipe 7: Olive and Herb Sourdough Bread

This rustic sourdough Sourdough is infused with savory flavors from olives and fresh herbs. It's perfect for dipping in olive oil or serving alongside a Mediterranean-inspired meal.

Prep Time: 30 minutes (active)

Cook Time: 45 minutes

Total Time: 12-14 hours (including fermentation and proofing)

Servings: 1 loaf (about 10-12 slices)

Ingredients:

- 400 grams Sourdough flour
- 100 grams whole wheat flour
- 350 grams water
- 100 grams active sourdough starter
- 10 grams sea salt
- 150 grams pitted olives, chopped
- 2 tablespoons chopped fresh rosemary or thyme
- 2 tablespoons olive oil (for drizzling)

Instructions:

Mix the Dough: In a large mixing bowl, combine the Sourdough flour, whole wheat flour, and water. Mix until fully combined and let it rest for 30 minutes (autolyse).

Add Starter and Salt: After the autolyse, mix in the sourdough starter and salt. Fold the dough onto itself until smooth.

Add Olives and Herbs: Gently fold the chopped olives and fresh herbs into the dough until evenly distributed.

Bulk Fermentation: Cover the dough and let it rise for 4-6 hours at room temperature. Perform stretch-and-folds every 30 minutes during the first 2 hours of fermentation.

Shaping: Shape the dough into a round or oval loaf. Place it in a floured proofing basket or a bowl lined with a towel and cover. Let it proof for 1-2 hours or refrigerate overnight.

Preheat the Oven: Preheat the oven to 450°F (230°C) with a Dutch oven inside.

Scoring and Baking: Score the dough with a sharp knife, then transfer it into the Dutch oven. Bake with the lid on for 20 minutes, then remove the lid and bake for an additional 20-25 minutes until golden brown and crisp.

Cooling: Drizzle with olive oil, allow the Sourdough to cool on a wire rack, and serve with more olive oil for dipping.

Recipe 8: Sourdough Oatmeal Bread

This hearty and slightly sweet Sourdough is made with oats for added fiber and a chewy texture. It's perfect for breakfast or as a snack topped with butter, honey, or jam.

Prep Time: 20 minutes (active)

Cook Time: 40 minutes

Total Time: 8-10 hours (including fermentation and proofing)

Servings: 1 loaf (about 10 slices)

Ingredients:

- 400 grams Sourdough flour
- 100 grams rolled oats (plus extra for topping)
- 350 grams water
- 100 grams active sourdough starter
- 10 grams sea salt
- 2 tablespoons honey or maple syrup

Instructions:

Mix the Dough: In a large bowl, combine the Sourdough flour, rolled oats, water, and honey or maple syrup. Mix until well combined and let it rest for 30 minutes (autolyse).

Add Starter and Salt: After the autolyse, mix in the sourdough starter and salt. Fold the dough until it becomes smooth and elastic.

Bulk Fermentation: Cover the dough and let it ferment at room temperature for 4-6 hours, performing stretch-and-folds every 30 minutes during the first 2 hours.

Shaping: Shape the dough into a loaf and place it in a proofing basket or bowl. Sprinkle extra oats on top for decoration.

Final Proof: Let the dough proof for 1-2 hours at room temperature or overnight in the refrigerator.

Preheat the Oven: Preheat the oven to 450°F (230°C) with a Dutch oven inside.

Scoring and Baking: Score the dough, transfer it to the Dutch oven, and bake for 20 minutes with the lid on. Remove the lid and bake for another 20-25 minutes until golden brown.

Cooling: Cool completely on a wire rack before slicing and serving.

Recipe 9: Walnut and Fig Sourdough Bread

This walnut and fig sourdough Sourdough combines the earthy, rich flavor of walnuts with the natural sweetness of dried figs. It's perfect for serving with cheese, butter, or honey and makes an excellent addition to a holiday table or as a sweet-savory snack.

Prep Time: 30 minutes (active)

Cook Time: 45 minutes

Total Time: 12-14 hours (including fermentation and proofing)

Servings: 1 loaf (about 12 slices)

Ingredients:

- 400 grams Sourdough flour
- 100 grams whole wheat flour
- 350 grams water
- 100 grams active sourdough starter
- 10 grams sea salt
- 150 grams dried figs, chopped
- 100 grams walnuts, roughly chopped
- 1 tablespoon honey (optional)

Instructions:

Prepare the Ingredients: In a small bowl, soak the dried figs in warm water for 30 minutes to soften them. Drain and set aside.

Mix the Dough: In a large mixing bowl, combine the Sourdough flour, whole wheat flour, and water. Mix until combined and let it rest for 30 minutes (autolyse).

Add Starter and Salt: After the autolyse, add the sourdough starter, salt, and honey (if using). Mix until well incorporated.

Fold in the Figs and Walnuts: Gently fold in the chopped figs and walnuts until they are evenly distributed throughout the dough.

Bulk Fermentation: Cover the dough and let it rise for 4-6 hours at room temperature, performing stretch-and-folds every 30 minutes during the first 2 hours to strengthen the dough.

Shaping: Shape the dough into a round or oval loaf. Place the shaped dough into a proofing basket or a bowl lined with a floured towel and cover. Let it proof at room temperature for 1-2 hours or refrigerate overnight.

Preheat the Oven: Preheat the oven to 450°F (230°C) with a Dutch oven inside.

Scoring and Baking: Score the top of the loaf and carefully transfer it to the preheated Dutch oven. Bake for 20 minutes with the lid on, then remove the lid and bake for an additional 25 minutes until the Sourdough is golden brown and crusty.

Cooling: Let the Sourdough cool completely on a wire rack before slicing.

Recipe 10: Sourdough Pumpkin Seed and Cranberry Bread

This flavorful Sourdough features the crunchy texture of pumpkin seeds and the sweet-tart burst of dried cranberries. It's a great loaf for fall or the holidays, pairing beautifully with soups or as a hearty breakfast option with butter or jam.

Prep Time: 25 minutes (active)

Cook Time: 45 minutes

Total Time: 10-12 hours (including fermentation and proofing)

Servings: 1 loaf (about 12 slices)

Ingredients:

- 400 grams Sourdough flour
- 100 grams whole wheat flour
- 350 grams water
- 100 grams active sourdough starter
- 10 grams sea salt
- 80 grams pumpkin seeds (plus extra for topping)
- 100 grams dried cranberries
- 1 tablespoon honey or maple syrup (optional)

Instructions:

Soak the Cranberries: Soak the dried cranberries in warm water for 20-30 minutes, then drain and set aside.

Mix the Dough: In a large bowl, combine the Sourdough flour, whole wheat flour, and water. Mix until fully combined and let it rest for 30 minutes (autolyse).

Add Starter and Salt: After the autolyse, mix in the sourdough starter, sea salt, and honey (if using). Fold the dough until it becomes smooth.

Incorporate the Seeds and Cranberries: Gently fold the pumpkin seeds and drained cranberries into the dough, ensuring they're evenly distributed.

Bulk Fermentation: Let the dough rise at room temperature for 4-6 hours, covering it and performing stretch-and-folds every 30 minutes during the first 2 hours.

Shaping: Shape the dough into a loaf and transfer it to a floured proofing basket or a bowl lined with a towel. Let it proof for 1-2 hours or overnight in the refrigerator.

Preheat the Oven: Preheat the oven to 450°F (230°C) with a Dutch oven inside.

Scoring and Baking: Score the dough and sprinkle extra pumpkin seeds on top before transferring the loaf to the Dutch oven. Bake with the lid on for 20 minutes, then remove the lid and bake for an additional 20-25 minutes until golden brown.

Cooling: Allow the loaf to cool on a wire rack before slicing and serving.

Recipe 11: Seeded Sourdough Rolls

These individual sourdough rolls are packed with a mix of seeds, making them crunchy on the outside and soft on the inside. They're perfect for sandwiches, burgers, or as dinner rolls, offering a nutrient boost thanks to the seeds.

Prep Time: 20 minutes (active)

Cook Time: 25 minutes

Total Time: 8-10 hours (including fermentation and proofing)

Servings: 12 rolls

Ingredients:

- 400 grams Sourdough flour
- 100 grams whole wheat flour

- 350 grams water
- 100 grams active sourdough starter
- 10 grams sea salt
- 30 grams sunflower seeds
- 20 grams sesame seeds
- 20 grams flaxseeds
- 20 grams pumpkin seeds

Instructions:

Prepare the Seeds: In a small bowl, mix the sunflower seeds, sesame seeds, flaxseeds, and pumpkin seeds. Set aside.

Mix the Dough: In a large mixing bowl, combine the Sourdough flour, whole wheat flour, and water. Mix until all the ingredients are fully combined, then let the dough rest for 30 minutes (autolyse).

Add Starter and Salt: After the autolyse, mix in the sourdough starter and sea salt. Fold the dough until smooth.

Incorporate the Seeds: Gently fold in the seed mixture, ensuring it's evenly distributed throughout the dough.

Bulk Fermentation: Cover the dough and let it rise at room temperature for 4-6 hours, performing stretch-and-folds every 30 minutes during the first 2 hours.

Shaping the Rolls: Divide the dough into 12 equal pieces and shape them into rolls. Place the rolls on a parchment-lined baking sheet and cover with a damp towel. Let them proof at room temperature for 1-2 hours or refrigerate overnight.

Preheat the Oven: Preheat the oven to 425°F (220°C).

Scoring and Baking: Score the tops of the rolls, then bake for 20-25 minutes until golden brown and firm on the outside.

Cooling: Allow the rolls to cool on a wire rack before serving.

Recipe 12: Sourdough Garlic and Herb Knots

These flavorful sourdough knots are perfect for serving as an appetizer or side dish. Infused with garlic and fresh herbs, they are soft, fragrant, and incredibly tasty, making them a great addition to a meal or as a snack.

Prep Time: 30 minutes (active)

Cook Time: 20 minutes

Total Time: 8-10 hours (including fermentation and proofing)

Servings: 12 knots

Ingredients:

- 400 grams Sourdough flour
- 100 grams whole wheat flour
- 350 grams water
- 100 grams active sourdough starter
- 10 grams sea salt
- 3 tablespoons olive oil
- 4 cloves garlic, minced
- 2 tablespoons chopped fresh rosemary or thyme
- 2 tablespoons fresh parsley, chopped (for garnish)

Instructions:

Mix the Dough: In a large bowl, combine the Sourdough flour, whole wheat flour, and water. Mix until well combined, then let the dough rest for 30 minutes (autolyse).

Add Starter and Salt: After the autolyse, add the sourdough starter, salt, and olive oil. Fold the dough until smooth and elastic.

Bulk Fermentation: Let the dough rise for 4-6 hours, covering it and performing stretch-and-folds every 30 minutes for the first 2 hours.

Shaping the Knots: Divide the dough into 12 equal pieces and roll each piece into a rope. Tie each rope into a knot and place them on a parchment-lined baking sheet. Cover with a towel and let them proof for 1-2 hours at room temperature.

Preheat the Oven: Preheat your oven to 425°F (220°C).

Prepare the Garlic and Herbs: In a small pan, gently heat the minced garlic and herbs in olive oil until fragrant. Brush the garlic and herb oil over the knots before baking.

Baking: Bake the knots for 18-20 minutes until golden brown.

Cooling and Garnishing: Once baked, brush the knots with any remaining garlic oil and sprinkle with fresh parsley. Serve warm.

These recipes showcase the diversity and versatility of sourdough baking, from simple loaves to more creative options like focaccia. Each recipe is designed to harness the power of natural fermentation and whole grains, offering not only delicious flavors but also substantial health benefits.

Chapter 6: Sourdough Bread Recipes for Healing

Sourdough bread is more than just a staple food—it can be a powerful tool for healing and maintaining health. By using nutrient-rich ingredients and traditional Sourdough -making techniques, we can create loaves that not only taste delicious but also nourish our bodies from the inside out. In this chapter, we focus on Sourdough s designed to enhance wellness, from supporting gut health to boosting immunity and providing sustainable energy.

Here, you'll find a collection of recipes that incorporate healing ingredients such as seeds, whole grains, herbs, and natural fermentation. These Sourdough s are perfect for those looking to improve their overall health through the power of real food.

Recipe 13: Immune-Boosting Sourdough with Garlic and Turmeric

Garlic and turmeric are well-known for their anti-inflammatory and immune-boosting properties. This golden-hued sourdough loaf combines these two superfoods into a delicious and healing

Sourdough that supports the body's natural defenses.

Prep Time: 25 minutes (active)

Cook Time: 45 minutes

Total Time: 10-12 hours (including fermentation and proofing)

Servings: 1 loaf (about 10-12 slices)

Ingredients:

- 400 grams Sourdough flour
- 100 grams whole wheat flour
- 350 grams water
- 100 grams active sourdough starter
- 10 grams sea salt
- 3 cloves garlic, minced
- 1 tablespoon ground turmeric
- 1 tablespoon olive oil (for greasing)
- Fresh cracked black pepper (optional, for topping)

Instructions:

Mix the Dough: In a large mixing bowl, combine the Sourdough flour, whole wheat flour, water, and turmeric. Mix until the ingredients are fully combined, then cover with a damp towel and let the dough rest for 30 minutes (autolyse).

Add Starter and Salt: After the autolyse, add the sourdough starter, sea salt, and minced garlic. Fold the dough onto itself until everything is well incorporated and the dough becomes smooth.

Bulk Fermentation: Cover the bowl and let the dough ferment at room temperature for 4-6 hours, performing stretch-and-folds every 30 minutes during the first 2 hours.

Shaping: Once the dough has risen, shape it into a round or oval loaf. Place it in a floured proofing basket or a bowl lined with a floured towel. Cover and let it proof for 1-2 hours at room temperature or overnight in the refrigerator.

Preheat the Oven: Preheat your oven to 450°F (230°C) with a Dutch oven inside.

Scoring and Baking: Before baking, score the top of the dough with a sharp knife and sprinkle cracked black pepper on top for an extra kick. Carefully transfer the dough to the preheated Dutch oven, cover with the lid, and bake for 20 minutes. Remove the lid and bake for another 25 minutes until the crust is golden brown.

Cooling: Transfer the Sourdough to a wire rack and allow it to cool completely before slicing and enjoying.

Recipe 14: Gut-Healing Sourdough with Fennel and Flaxseeds

This gut-friendly loaf is packed with fennel seeds, known for their digestive benefits, and flaxseeds, which are rich in omega-3 fatty acids and fiber. It's an excellent Sourdough for those looking to support their digestive health while enjoying a flavorful, crunchy loaf.

Prep Time: 30 minutes (active)

Cook Time: 40 minutes

Total Time: 10-12 hours (including fermentation and proofing)

Servings: 1 loaf (about 12 slices)

Ingredients:

- 400 grams whole wheat flour
- 100 grams Sourdough flour
- 350 grams water
- 100 grams active sourdough starter

- 10 grams sea salt
- 2 tablespoons flaxseeds
- 1 tablespoon fennel seeds
- 1 tablespoon olive oil (optional)

Instructions:

Prepare the Seeds: In a small bowl, soak the flaxseeds and fennel seeds in 50 grams of water for about 30 minutes.

Mix the Dough: In a large bowl, combine the whole wheat flour, Sourdough flour, and remaining water. Mix until combined and let the dough rest for 30 minutes (autolyse).

Add Starter, Salt, and Seeds: After the autolyse, add the sourdough starter, sea salt, and the soaked seeds (along with their soaking water). Fold the dough until everything is well incorporated.

Bulk Fermentation: Cover the dough and let it rise for 4-6 hours, performing stretch-and-folds every 30 minutes for the first 2 hours.

Shaping: Shape the dough into a round or oval loaf. Place it in a proofing basket or bowl lined with a floured towel and cover. Let the dough proof at room temperature for 1-2 hours or overnight in the refrigerator.

Preheat the Oven: Preheat your oven to 450°F (230°C) with a Dutch oven inside.

Scoring and Baking: Score the top of the dough and carefully transfer it to the Dutch oven. Bake with the lid on for 20 minutes, then remove the lid and bake for another 20 minutes until the crust is crisp and golden.

Cooling: Let the Sourdough cool on a wire rack before slicing.

Recipe 15: Energy-Boosting Multigrain Sourdough

Packed with a variety of whole grains and seeds, this multigrain sourdough provides sustained energy and is perfect for fueling active lifestyles. The combination of grains adds texture, flavor, and a host of nutrients, making this loaf a wholesome choice for breakfast or as a pre-workout snack.

Prep Time: 30 minutes (active)

Cook Time: 45 minutes

Total Time: 12-14 hours (including fermentation and proofing)

Servings: 1 loaf (about 12 slices)

Ingredients:

- 200 grams whole wheat flour
- 200 grams Sourdough flour
- 50 grams rolled oats
- 50 grams millet or quinoa (cooked and cooled)
- 350 grams water
- 100 grams active sourdough starter
- 10 grams sea salt
- 30 grams sunflower seeds
- 30 grams flaxseeds
- 30 grams sesame seeds

Instructions:

Prepare the Grains: Cook the millet or quinoa according to package instructions, then allow it to cool. In a separate bowl, soak the rolled oats and seeds in 50 grams of water for 30 minutes.

Mix the Dough: In a large mixing bowl, combine the whole wheat flour, Sourdough flour, and water. Mix until fully incorporated and let the dough rest for 30 minutes (autolyse).

Add Starter and Salt: After the autolyse, mix in the sourdough starter, sea salt, cooked millet or quinoa, and the soaked oats and seeds. Fold the dough until smooth and elastic.

Bulk Fermentation: Cover the dough and let it rise at room temperature for 4-6 hours, performing stretch-and-folds every 30 minutes during the first 2 hours.

Shaping: Shape the dough into a round loaf and place it into a floured proofing basket or a bowl lined with a towel. Cover and proof at room temperature for 1-2 hours or overnight in the refrigerator.

Preheat the Oven: Preheat the oven to 450°F (230°C) with a Dutch oven inside.

Scoring and Baking: Score the dough, then transfer it to the preheated Dutch oven. Bake with the lid on for 20 minutes, then remove the lid and bake for another 25 minutes until the crust is golden and firm.

Cooling: Allow the Sourdough to cool on a wire rack before slicing.

Recipe 16: Anti-Inflammatory Sourdough with Ginger and Turmeric

Both ginger and turmeric are powerful anti-inflammatory spices. This sourdough loaf incorporates these healing ingredients to create a bright, flavorful Sourdough that supports overall health and reduces inflammation in the body. It's great for pairing with soups or as a unique sandwich Sourdough .

Prep Time: 25 minutes (active)

Cook Time: 45 minutes

Total Time: 10-12 hours (including fermentation and proofing)

Servings: 1 loaf (about 10-12 slices)

Ingredients:

- 400 grams Sourdough flour
- 100 grams whole wheat flour
- 350 grams water
- 100 grams active sourdough starter
- 10 grams sea salt
- 2 tablespoons ground turmeric
- 1 tablespoon freshly grated ginger
- 1 tablespoon honey or maple syrup (optional)

Instructions:

Mix the Dough: In a large bowl, combine the Sourdough flour, whole wheat flour, turmeric, and water. Mix until well combined and let the dough rest for 30 minutes (autolyse).

Add Starter and Salt: After the autolyse, add the sourdough starter, sea salt, and grated ginger. Mix the dough until smooth and elastic. If desired, add honey or maple syrup for a slightly sweet note.

Bulk Fermentation: Cover the dough and let it rise at room temperature for 4-6 hours, performing stretch-and-folds every 30 minutes during the first 2 hours.

Shaping: Shape the dough into a round loaf and place it into a floured proofing basket or a bowl lined with a floured towel. Cover and proof at room temperature for 1-2 hours or refrigerate overnight.

Preheat the Oven: Preheat your oven to 450°F (230°C) with a Dutch oven inside.

Scoring and Baking: Score the top of the dough with a sharp knife, then transfer the dough to the Dutch oven. Bake with the lid on for 20 minutes, then remove the lid and bake for another 25 minutes until the crust is golden brown.

Cooling: Let the loaf cool completely on a wire rack before slicing.

Recipe 17: Omega-3 Rich Sourdough with Chia and Flaxseeds

This Sourdough is designed to deliver a healthy dose of omega-3 fatty acids, which are important for heart health and reducing inflammation. The combination of chia and flaxseeds adds a nutty flavor and a crunchy texture, making this loaf a nutritious addition to any meal.

Prep Time: 25 minutes (active)

Cook Time: 40 minutes

Total Time: 10-12 hours (including fermentation and proofing)

Servings: 1 loaf (about 10 slices)

Ingredients:

- 400 grams Sourdough flour
- 100 grams whole wheat flour
- 350 grams water
- 100 grams active sourdough starter
- 10 grams sea salt
- 2 tablespoons chia seeds
- 2 tablespoons flaxseeds

Instructions:

Soak the Seeds: In a small bowl, soak the chia seeds and flaxseeds in 50 grams of water for 30 minutes.

Mix the Dough: In a large bowl, combine the Sourdough flour, whole wheat flour, and remaining water. Mix until combined and let the dough rest for 30 minutes (autolyse).

Add Starter, Salt, and Seeds: Add the sourdough starter, sea salt, and the soaked seeds to the dough. Fold the dough until smooth and elastic.

Bulk Fermentation: Cover the dough and let it ferment for 4-6 hours, performing stretch-and-folds every 30 minutes during the first 2 hours.

Shaping: Shape the dough into a loaf and place it into a proofing basket or a bowl lined with a towel. Cover and proof for 1-2 hours or overnight in the refrigerator.

Preheat the Oven: Preheat the oven to 450°F (230°C) with a Dutch oven inside.

Scoring and Baking: Score the dough and transfer it to the Dutch oven. Bake with the lid on for 20 minutes, then remove the lid and bake for another 20-25 minutes until golden brown.

Cooling: Cool completely on a wire rack before slicing.

Recipe 18: Vitamin C-Rich Sourdough with Citrus and Sunflower Seeds

This bright and zesty loaf is packed with the immune-boosting benefits of citrus zest, which is high in vitamin C and antioxidants. The addition of sunflower seeds provides a dose of healthy fats and vitamin E, making this Sourdough a nutrient-dense choice for boosting immunity.

Prep Time: 30 minutes (active)

Cook Time: 45 minutes

Total Time: 12-14 hours (including fermentation and proofing)

Servings: 1 loaf (about 10-12 slices)

Ingredients:

- 400 grams Sourdough flour
- 100 grams whole wheat flour
- 350 grams water
- 100 grams active sourdough starter
- 10 grams sea salt
- Zest of 1 orange
- Zest of 1 lemon

- 50 grams sunflower seeds (plus extra for topping)
- 1 tablespoon honey or maple syrup (optional)

Instructions:

Prepare the Zest: Grate the zest from one orange and one lemon. Set aside.

Mix the Dough: In a large bowl, combine the Sourdough flour, whole wheat flour, and water. Mix until the ingredients are fully combined and let the dough rest for 30 minutes (autolyse).

Add Starter, Salt, and Zest: After the autolyse, add the sourdough starter, sea salt, citrus zest, and honey (if using). Mix the dough until smooth and elastic.

Fold in the Seeds: Gently fold the sunflower seeds into the dough until they are evenly distributed.

Bulk Fermentation: Cover the dough and let it rise at room temperature for 4-6 hours, performing stretch-and-folds every 30 minutes for the first 2 hours.

Shaping: Shape the dough into a round or oval loaf. Place it into a proofing basket or bowl lined with a floured towel. Let it proof at room temperature for 1-2 hours, or refrigerate overnight.

Preheat the Oven: Preheat your oven to 450°F (230°C) with a Dutch oven inside.

Scoring and Baking: Score the top of the loaf with a sharp knife, sprinkle with extra sunflower seeds, and carefully transfer the dough to the preheated Dutch oven. Bake for 20 minutes with the lid on, then remove the lid and bake for another 25 minutes until the crust is golden brown and fragrant.

Cooling: Transfer the Sourdough to a wire rack and let it cool completely before slicing.

Recipe 19: Sourdough Beetroot Bread

Beetroot is known for its anti-inflammatory properties and ability to improve blood circulation. This beautiful pink-hued loaf is not only visually striking but also packed with nutrients that support heart health and provide antioxidants.

Prep Time: 30 minutes (active)

Cook Time: 45 minutes

Total Time: 12-14 hours (including fermentation and proofing)

Servings: 1 loaf (about 12 slices)

Ingredients:

- 400 grams Sourdough flour
- 100 grams whole wheat flour
- 350 grams water
- 100 grams active sourdough starter
- 10 grams sea salt
- 150 grams roasted beets, pureed
- 2 tablespoons olive oil (optional)
- 1 tablespoon honey or maple syrup (optional)

Instructions:

Prepare the Beets: Roast the beets in the oven at 400°F (200°C) for about 30-40 minutes until tender. Let them cool, then peel and puree in a food processor. Set aside.

Mix the Dough: In a large mixing bowl, combine the Sourdough flour, whole wheat flour, water, and pureed beets. Mix until combined, then let the dough rest for 30 minutes (autolyse).

Add Starter, Salt, and Olive Oil: After the autolyse, add the sourdough starter, sea salt, and olive oil (if using). Mix until smooth and elastic.

Bulk Fermentation: Cover the dough and let it rise at room temperature for 4-6 hours, performing stretch-and-folds every 30 minutes during the first 2 hours.

Shaping: Shape the dough into a loaf and place it in a floured proofing basket or a bowl lined with a towel. Let the dough proof for 1-2 hours at room temperature, or refrigerate overnight.

Preheat the Oven: Preheat the oven to 450°F (230°C) with a Dutch oven inside.

Scoring and Baking: Score the dough and transfer it to the preheated Dutch oven. Bake for 20 minutes with the lid on, then remove the lid and bake for another 20-25 minutes until the crust is golden brown and the Sourdough is baked through.

Cooling: Cool the loaf on a wire rack before slicing and serving.

Recipe 20: Protein-Rich Sourdough with Hemp and Chia Seeds

Hemp and chia seeds are excellent sources of plant-based protein and omega-3 fatty acids, making this loaf ideal for those looking to boost their protein intake. This Sourdough is perfect for athletes, fitness enthusiasts, or anyone seeking a nutrient-dense, protein-rich Sourdough .

Prep Time: 25 minutes (active)

Cook Time: 45 minutes

Total Time: 10-12 hours (including fermentation and proofing)

Servings: 1 loaf (about 12 slices)

Ingredients:

- 400 grams Sourdough flour
- 100 grams whole wheat flour
- 350 grams water
- 100 grams active sourdough starter
- 10 grams sea salt
- 2 tablespoons hemp seeds
- 2 tablespoons chia seeds
- 1 tablespoon honey or maple syrup (optional)

Instructions:

Prepare the Seeds: In a small bowl, soak the chia seeds and hemp seeds in 50 grams of water for 30 minutes to hydrate.

Mix the Dough: In a large bowl, combine the Sourdough flour, whole wheat flour, and remaining water. Mix until fully incorporated and let it rest for 30 minutes (autolyse).

Add Starter, Salt, and Seeds: After the autolyse, mix in the sourdough starter, sea salt, and the soaked seeds. Fold the dough until smooth and elastic.

Bulk Fermentation: Let the dough rise for 4-6 hours, performing stretch-and-folds every 30 minutes during the first 2 hours.

Shaping: Shape the dough into a loaf and place it into a proofing basket or a bowl lined with a floured towel. Let the dough proof at room temperature for 1-2 hours or overnight in the refrigerator.

Preheat the Oven: Preheat the oven to 450°F (230°C) with a Dutch oven inside.

Scoring and Baking: Score the loaf and carefully transfer it to the Dutch oven. Bake with the lid on for 20 minutes, then remove the lid and bake for another 20-25 minutes until golden brown.

Cooling: Cool completely on a wire rack before slicing.

Recipe 21: Sourdough with Spirulina and Pumpkin Seeds

Spirulina is a nutrient-dense algae that's high in protein, vitamins, and minerals, making it a powerful superfood addition to any Sourdough . Paired with pumpkin seeds, which are rich in magnesium and antioxidants, this Sourdough is great for supporting overall wellness and reducing inflammation.

Prep Time: 30 minutes (active)

Cook Time: 40 minutes

Total Time: 12-14 hours (including fermentation and proofing)

Servings: 1 loaf (about 10 slices)

Ingredients:

- 400 grams Sourdough flour
- 100 grams whole wheat flour
- 350 grams water
- 100 grams active sourdough starter
- 10 grams sea salt
- 1 tablespoon spirulina powder
- 50 grams pumpkin seeds (plus extra for topping)

Instructions:

Mix the Dough: In a large bowl, combine the Sourdough flour, whole wheat flour, spirulina powder, and water. Mix until combined, then let the dough rest for 30 minutes (autolyse).

Add Starter, Salt, and Pumpkin Seeds: After the autolyse, add the sourdough starter, sea salt, and pumpkin seeds. Fold the dough until smooth and elastic.

Bulk Fermentation: Cover the dough and let it rise at room temperature for 4-6 hours, performing stretch-and-folds every 30 minutes during the first 2 hours.

Shaping: Shape the dough into a round loaf and place it into a floured proofing basket or a bowl lined with a towel. Cover and proof at room temperature for 1-2 hours, or refrigerate overnight.

Preheat the Oven: Preheat your oven to 450°F (230°C) with a Dutch oven inside.

Scoring and Baking: Score the loaf and transfer it to the preheated Dutch oven. Bake with the lid on for 20 minutes, then remove the lid and bake for another 20-25 minutes until golden brown and firm.

Cooling: Let the loaf cool completely before slicing and serving.

Recipe 22: Detox Sourdough with Activated Charcoal and Sesame Seeds

Activated charcoal is known for its detoxifying properties, and while it's subtle in flavor, it gives this Sourdough a striking black color. Paired with sesame seeds, which provide antioxidants and healthy fats, this loaf is as nutritious as it is unique.

Prep Time: 25 minutes (active)

Cook Time: 45 minutes

Total Time: 12-14 hours (including fermentation and proofing)

Servings: 1 loaf (about 10-12 slices)

Ingredients:

- 400 grams Sourdough flour
- 100 grams whole wheat flour
- 350 grams water
- 100 grams active sourdough starter
- 10 grams sea salt
- 2 teaspoons activated charcoal powder

- 50 grams black sesame seeds (plus extra for topping)

Instructions:

Mix the Dough: In a large bowl, combine the Sourdough flour, whole wheat flour, activated charcoal powder, and water. Mix until combined, then let the dough rest for 30 minutes (autolyse).

Add Starter, Salt, and Sesame Seeds: After the autolyse, mix in the sourdough starter, sea salt, and sesame seeds. Fold the dough until smooth and elastic.

Bulk Fermentation: Let the dough rise at room temperature for 4-6 hours, performing stretch-and-folds every 30 minutes for the first 2 hours.

Shaping: Shape the dough into a loaf and place it into a floured proofing basket or a bowl lined with a towel. Let it proof at room temperature for 1-2 hours, or refrigerate overnight.

Preheat the Oven: Preheat the oven to 450°F (230°C) with a Dutch oven inside.

Scoring and Baking: Score the loaf and transfer it to the Dutch oven. Bake with the lid on for 20 minutes, then remove the lid and bake for another 20-25 minutes until firm and golden.

Cooling: Allow the Sourdough to cool completely on a wire rack before slicing.

These healing Sourdough recipes are designed to enhance wellness through the power of whole grains, seeds, and natural fermentation. Whether you're boosting your immune system, supporting digestion, or simply fueling your body with nutritious ingredients, these loaves are crafted to help you feel healthier, younger, and stronger every day.

Chapter 7: Baking for All Ages and Needs

Sourdough bread is a universal food, beloved by people of all ages. However, different age groups and lifestyles have unique nutritional needs that can be supported by carefully crafted sourdough recipes. Whether you're baking for growing children, active adults, or seniors looking to maintain strength and vitality, sourdough can be tailored to suit everyone's health needs.

This chapter provides sourdough recipes designed with specific dietary requirements in mind. From kid-friendly loaves to nutrient-dense options for athletes and gentle recipes for seniors, these sourdough s provide a balanced, wholesome way to support health at every stage of life.

Recipe 23: Kid-Friendly Sourdough with Oats and Honey

This soft, slightly sweet sourdough is perfect for children. The oats add fiber and nutrition, while a touch of honey provides natural sweetness. It's great for school lunches, toast, or as a base for a healthy sandwich.

Prep Time: 20 minutes (active)

Cook Time: 35 minutes

Total Time: 8-10 hours (including fermentation and proofing)

Servings: 1 loaf (about 12 slices)

Ingredients:

- 400 grams bread flour
- 100 grams rolled oats (plus extra for topping)
- 350 grams water
- 100 grams active sourdough starter
- 10 grams sea salt
- 2 tablespoons honey
- 1 tablespoon olive oil (optional)

Instructions:

Prepare the Oats: Soak the oats in 50 grams of the water for 30 minutes to soften them.

Mix the Dough: In a large bowl, combine the bread flour, remaining water, honey, and olive oil (if using). Mix until fully combined, then let the dough rest for 30 minutes (autolyse).

Add Starter, Salt, and Oats: After the autolyse, mix in the sourdough starter, sea salt, and soaked oats. Fold the dough until smooth.

Bulk Fermentation: Let the dough rise at room temperature for 4-6 hours, performing stretch-and-folds every 30 minutes for the first 2 hours.

Shaping: Shape the dough into a loaf and place it into a proofing basket or bowl lined with a floured towel. Let it proof for 1-2 hours at room temperature, or refrigerate overnight.

Preheat the Oven: Preheat the oven to 425°F (220°C) with a Dutch oven inside.

Scoring and Baking: Score the dough and transfer it to the Dutch oven. Sprinkle extra oats on top. Bake with the lid on for 20 minutes, then remove the lid and bake for another 15 minutes until golden brown.

Cooling: Cool the Sourdough on a wire rack before slicing.

Recipe 24: Soft Sourdough Bread for Seniors with Flaxseeds

This gentle sourdough loaf is designed for seniors who may prefer softer textures while still benefiting from nutrient-rich ingredients like flaxseeds, which support digestion and cardiovascular health. The Sourdough is easy to chew and digest, making it ideal for older adults.

Prep Time: 20 minutes (active)

Cook Time: 40 minutes

Total Time: 10-12 hours (including fermentation and proofing)

Servings: 1 loaf (about 10-12 slices)

Ingredients:

- 400 grams bread flour
- 100 grams whole wheat flour
- 350 grams water
- 100 grams active sourdough starter
- 10 grams sea salt
- 2 tablespoons flaxseeds
- 1 tablespoon olive oil (optional)

Instructions:

Prepare the Flaxseeds: Soak the flaxseeds in 50 grams of water for 30 minutes to soften.

Mix the Dough: In a large bowl, combine the Sourdough flour, whole wheat flour, remaining water, and olive oil (if using). Mix until fully incorporated, then let the dough rest for 30 minutes (autolyse).

Add Starter, Salt, and Seeds: After the autolyse, mix in the sourdough starter, sea salt, and soaked flaxseeds. Fold the dough until smooth and elastic.

Bulk Fermentation: Let the dough rise for 4-6 hours at room temperature, performing stretch-and-folds every 30 minutes during the first 2 hours.

Shaping: Shape the dough into a round or oval loaf and place it into a proofing basket or bowl lined with a floured towel. Let it proof for 1-2 hours, or refrigerate overnight.

Preheat the Oven: Preheat the oven to 425°F (220°C) with a Dutch oven inside.

Scoring and Baking: Score the dough, then transfer it to the Dutch oven. Bake with the lid on for 20 minutes, then remove the lid and bake for another 20 minutes until golden brown.

Cooling: Cool the loaf on a wire rack before slicing and serving.

Recipe 25: High-Protein Sourdough for Athletes with Quinoa and Seeds

Athletes need a high-protein, nutrient-dense Sourdough to fuel their bodies. This loaf incorporates quinoa and a variety of seeds, providing sustained energy, protein, and healthy fats to support an active lifestyle.

Prep Time: 30 minutes (active)

Cook Time: 45 minutes

Total Time: 12-14 hours (including fermentation and proofing)

Servings: 1 loaf (about 12 slices)

Ingredients:

- 400 grams bread flour
- 100 grams cooked quinoa (cooled)
- 350 grams water
- 100 grams active sourdough starter
- 10 grams sea salt
- 2 tablespoons sunflower seeds
- 2 tablespoons chia seeds
- 2 tablespoons flaxseeds

Instructions:

Prepare the Quinoa and Seeds: Cook the quinoa according to package instructions and allow it to cool. Soak the sunflower seeds, chia seeds, and flaxseeds in 50 grams of water for 30 minutes.

Mix the Dough: In a large bowl, combine the Sourdough flour, remaining water, and cooked quinoa. Mix until well combined, then let the dough rest for 30 minutes (autolyse).

Add Starter, Salt, and Seeds: After the autolyse, mix in the sourdough starter, sea salt, and soaked seeds. Fold the dough until smooth.

Bulk Fermentation: Cover the dough and let it rise for 4-6 hours at room temperature, performing stretch-and-folds every 30 minutes for the first 2 hours.

Shaping: Shape the dough into a loaf and place it into a floured proofing basket or a bowl lined with a towel. Let the dough proof for 1-2 hours at room temperature or refrigerate overnight.

Preheat the Oven: Preheat your oven to 450°F (230°C) with a Dutch oven inside.

Scoring and Baking: Score the dough and carefully transfer it to the Dutch oven. Bake for 20 minutes with the lid on, then remove the lid and bake for another 25 minutes until the crust is firm and golden.

Cooling: Cool the Sourdough on a wire rack before slicing and serving.

Recipe 26: Gluten-Free Sourdough with Buckwheat and Teff

For those with gluten sensitivities, this gluten-free sourdough uses buckwheat and teff flour, both naturally gluten-free grains. This hearty loaf is high in fiber and protein, providing a healthy alternative for those avoiding gluten.

Prep Time: 25 minutes (active)

Cook Time: 50 minutes

Total Time: 12-14 hours (including fermentation and proofing)

Servings: 1 loaf (about 10-12 slices)

Ingredients:

- 200 grams buckwheat flour
- 200 grams teff flour
- 350 grams water

- 100 grams gluten-free sourdough starter
- 10 grams sea salt
- 1 tablespoon psyllium husk (for structure)
- 2 tablespoons olive oil

Instructions:

Mix the Dough: In a large bowl, combine the buckwheat flour, teff flour, psyllium husk, and water. Mix until fully incorporated and let the dough rest for 30 minutes (autolyse).

Add Starter and Salt: After the autolyse, mix in the gluten-free sourdough starter, sea salt, and olive oil. Stir well until the dough is smooth and thick.

Bulk Fermentation: Cover the dough and let it rise at room temperature for 4-6 hours.

Shaping: Shape the dough into a round or oval loaf and place it into a greased proofing basket or a bowl lined with a towel. Let it proof for 1-2 hours at room temperature or refrigerate overnight.

Preheat the Oven: Preheat the oven to 425°F (220°C) with a Dutch oven inside.

Scoring and Baking: Score the dough and carefully transfer it to the Dutch oven. Bake with the lid on for 25 minutes, then remove the lid and bake for another 25 minutes until golden brown and cooked through.

Cooling: Cool the gluten-free Sourdough on a wire rack before slicing.

Recipe 27: Nut-Free Sourdough for Kids

This nut-free sourdough is perfect for children with nut allergies. It's soft, fluffy, and safe for school lunches or snacks. The loaf is slightly sweet, making it appealing to even the pickiest eaters.

Prep Time: 20 minutes (active)

Cook Time: 35 minutes

Total Time: 8-10 hours (including fermentation and proofing)

Servings: 1 loaf (about 12 slices)

Ingredients:

- 400 grams bread flour
- 100 grams whole wheat flour
- 350 grams water
- 100 grams active sourdough starter
- 10 grams sea salt

- 2 tablespoons honey or maple syrup (optional)

Instructions:

Mix the Dough: In a large bowl, combine the Sourdough flour, whole wheat flour, water, and honey or maple syrup (if using). Mix until fully combined, then let the dough rest for 30 minutes (autolyse).

Add Starter and Salt: After the autolyse, mix in the sourdough starter and sea salt. Fold the dough until it becomes smooth and elastic.

Bulk Fermentation: Let the dough rise for 4-6 hours at room temperature, performing stretch-and-folds every 30 minutes for the first 2 hours.

Shaping: Shape the dough into a loaf and place it into a proofing basket or a bowl lined with a floured towel. Let it proof for 1-2 hours at room temperature, or refrigerate overnight.

Preheat the Oven: Preheat the oven to 425°F (220°C) with a Dutch oven inside.

Scoring and Baking: Score the dough and transfer it to the preheated Dutch oven. Bake for 20 minutes with the lid on, then remove the lid and bake for another 15 minutes until golden brown.

Cooling: Cool the bread completely on a wire rack before slicing and serving.

These recipes offer something for everyone, from children to seniors and athletes to those with gluten sensitivities or nut allergies. With thoughtful ingredients and careful preparation, these sourdoughs nourish the body and support a healthy, balanced lifestyle at every age.

Chapter 8: Real Sourdough, Real Life

Sourdough has long been a symbol of nourishment, comfort, and community. When you bake real Sourdough at home, you're not just feeding your body; you're connecting with tradition and creating something to share with others. Real sourdough has the power to bring people together, whether it's a simple loaf shared at a family dinner or an intricate sourdough creation served at a special event.

In this chapter, we explore how to make real sourdough a part of your everyday life and how to build a sustainable sourdough -baking routine. Whether you're baking for yourself, your family, or your community, these recipes and tips will help you infuse each day with the healing power of real sourdough.

Building a Healing Sourdough Routine

The key to reaping the health benefits of real sourdough lies in making it a regular part of your diet. By incorporating naturally leavened, whole grain sourdough into your meals, you can create a consistent source of nourishment that supports your physical and mental well-being.

1. Meal Planning with Sourdough

Planning your meals around real Sourdough is a simple way to ensure that it becomes a staple in your home. Here are a few ideas for integrating Sourdough into daily meals:

Breakfast: A slice of toasted sourdough with avocado, eggs, or nut butter makes for a nutritious and satisfying start to the day.

Lunch: Use your homemade sourdough as the base for sandwiches, paired with fresh vegetables, hummus, or lean proteins.

Dinner: Serve sourdough alongside soups, stews, or salads to round out your meal with complex carbohydrates and fiber.

Snacks: Real sourdough can be transformed into healthy snacks, from bruschetta topped with tomatoes and herbs to garlic Sourdough with olive oil and sea salt.

2. Time-Saving Tips for Sourdough Baking

One of the challenges of baking real sourdough is finding the time to fit it into your busy schedule. However, with a few time-saving strategies, you can bake fresh loaves without dedicating your entire day to the process.

Autolyse Overnight: Start the dough in the evening by mixing the flour and water, allowing it to autolyse overnight. In the morning, simply add your sourdough starter and salt, and the dough is ready for bulk fermentation.

Refrigerate for Flavor: After shaping your dough, refrigerate it for 12-24 hours to develop a deeper flavor and extend the fermentation time. This way, you can bake the sourdough when it's convenient for you.

Bake in Batches: If you have the time and oven space, bake multiple loaves at once. Sourdough freezes well, so you can store extra loaves for later use.

Recipe 28: Celebration Sourdough with Dried Fruit and Nuts

This special-occasion sourdough is perfect for holidays, birthdays, or any celebration. The combination of dried fruit and nuts makes this loaf rich in flavor, while the natural fermentation process gives it a soft, chewy texture. It's a wonderful sourdough to serve with cheese, jams, or simply on its own.

Prep Time: 30 minutes (active)

Cook Time: 45 minutes

Total Time: 12-14 hours (including fermentation and proofing)

Servings: 1 large loaf (about 14 slices)

Ingredients:

- 400 grams Sourdough flour
- 100 grams whole wheat flour
- 350 grams water
- 100 grams active sourdough starter
- 10 grams sea salt
- 100 grams dried figs (or any dried fruit), chopped
- 100 grams walnuts (or any nut), roughly chopped
- 2 tablespoons honey or maple syrup (optional)

Instructions:

Prepare the Fruit and Nuts: In a small bowl, soak the dried figs in warm water for 30 minutes. Drain and set aside. Chop the walnuts roughly and set aside as well.

Mix the Dough: In a large bowl, combine the Sourdough flour, whole wheat flour, and water.

Mix until fully incorporated and let it rest for 30 minutes (autolyse).

Add Starter, Salt, Fruit, and Nuts: After the autolyse, mix in the sourdough starter, sea salt, soaked dried fruit, and walnuts. Fold the dough until everything is well distributed.

Bulk Fermentation: Cover the dough and let it rise for 4-6 hours, performing stretch-and-folds every 30 minutes for the first 2 hours.

Shaping: Shape the dough into a round loaf and place it into a proofing basket or a bowl lined with a floured towel. Let it proof at room temperature for 1-2 hours, or refrigerate overnight.

Preheat the Oven: Preheat the oven to 450°F (230°C) with a Dutch oven inside.

Scoring and Baking: Score the top of the dough with a sharp knife and carefully transfer it to the Dutch oven. Bake for 20 minutes with the lid on, then remove the lid and bake for another 25 minutes until the crust is golden brown and firm.

Cooling: Let the loaf cool completely before slicing and serving at your next celebration.

Recipe 29: Sourdough Focaccia for Sharing

Focaccia is a simple yet versatile sourdough that's perfect for sharing with family and friends. This sourdough version is infused with olive oil and herbs, making it the ideal accompaniment to soups, salads, or as an appetizer at gatherings.

Prep Time: 20 minutes (active)

Cook Time: 25 minutes

Total Time: 8-10 hours (including fermentation and proofing)

Servings: 1 large focaccia (about 12 pieces)

Ingredients:

- 450 grams Sourdough flour
- 350 grams water
- 100 grams active sourdough starter
- 10 grams sea salt
- 4 tablespoons olive oil (plus extra for drizzling)
- Fresh rosemary or thyme (optional)
- Flaky sea salt (for topping)

Instructions:

Mix the Dough: In a large bowl, combine the Sourdough flour, water, and sourdough starter. Mix until all ingredients are combined, then let the dough rest for 30 minutes (autolyse).

Add Salt and Olive Oil: After the autolyse, mix in the sea salt and 2 tablespoons of olive oil. Gently fold the dough until smooth.

Bulk Fermentation: Let the dough rise for 4-6 hours at room temperature, performing stretch-and-folds every 30 minutes for the first 2 hours.

Shaping and Proofing: Once the dough has risen, generously oil a baking tray or cast iron skillet. Turn the dough out onto the tray and gently stretch it to fit the tray. Cover with a damp towel and let it proof for 1-2 hours.

Preheat the Oven: Preheat the oven to 450°F (230°C).

Topping and Baking: Before baking, drizzle the dough with more olive oil and sprinkle with rosemary, thyme, and flaky sea salt. Press your fingers into the dough to create dimples. Bake for 20-25 minutes until golden brown.

Cooling: Let the focaccia cool slightly before cutting into squares and serving warm. It's perfect for sharing at dinner parties or family meals.

Recipe 30: Sourdough Pizza Dough for Family Night

This sourdough pizza dough is a fun way to get the family involved in cooking. It's chewy, flavorful, and can be topped with anything from classic margherita ingredients to creative combinations. This recipe makes enough dough for two pizzas, perfect for a family pizza night.

Prep Time: 20 minutes (active)

Cook Time: 12-15 minutes (per pizza)

Total Time: 8-10 hours (including fermentation and proofing)

Servings: 2 large pizzas

Ingredients:

- 400 grams Sourdough flour
- 300 grams water
- 100 grams active sourdough starter
- 10 grams sea salt

- 2 tablespoons olive oil (optional)

Instructions:

Mix the Dough: In a large bowl, combine the Sourdough flour, water, and sourdough starter. Mix until fully combined, then let the dough rest for 30 minutes (autolyse).

Add Salt and Olive Oil: After the autolyse, add the sea salt and olive oil (if using). Fold the dough until smooth and elastic.

Bulk Fermentation: Cover the dough and let it rise for 4-6 hours at room temperature, performing stretch-and-folds every 30 minutes during the first 2 hours.

Divide and Proof: After bulk fermentation, divide the dough into two equal portions. Shape each portion into a ball and place them on a floured surface. Cover with a towel and let them proof for 1-2 hours.

Preheat the Oven: Preheat your oven to 475°F (245°C). If you have a pizza stone, place it in the oven to preheat as well.

Shaping and Topping: Roll out each portion of dough into a thin round. Top with your favorite pizza sauce, cheese, and toppings.

Baking: Bake each pizza for 12-15 minutes, until the crust is golden and the toppings are bubbly.

Serving: Slice and serve hot for a fun family meal.

Recipe 31: Sourdough Flatbreads for Quick Meals

Sourdough flatbreads are quick, versatile, and can be used in a variety of ways. Whether you use them as a wrap, a base for pizza, or served with dips, these flatSourdough s are soft, flavorful, and easy to make.

Prep Time: 10 minutes (active)

Cook Time: 10 minutes (per flatSourdough)

Total Time: 6-8 hours (including fermentation and proofing)

Servings: 8 flatSourdough s

Ingredients:

- 300 grams Sourdough flour
- 100 grams whole wheat flour
- 250 grams water
- 100 grams active sourdough starter
- 10 grams sea salt

- 2 tablespoons olive oil (optional)

Instructions:

Mix the Dough: In a large mixing bowl, combine the bread flour, whole wheat flour, water, and sourdough starter. Mix until everything is combined and let it rest for 30 minutes (autolyse).

Add Salt and Oil: After the autolyse, add the sea salt and olive oil. Fold the dough until smooth.

Bulk Fermentation: Let the dough rise at room temperature for 4-6 hours.

Divide and Shape: After the dough has risen, divide it into 8 equal portions. Roll each portion into a ball, then flatten each ball into a round flatbread about ¼ inch thick.

Preheat the Skillet: Preheat a cast iron skillet or non-stick pan over medium-high heat.

Cooking the Flatbreads: Cook each flatSourdough in the skillet for 2-3 minutes on each side until lightly browned and cooked through. Brush with olive oil if desired.

Serving: Serve warm with dips, or use them as wraps for sandwiches.

Recipe 32: Rustic Sourdough Rolls for Gatherings

These rustic sourdough rolls are perfect for family dinners, holidays, or gatherings with friends. They have a soft crumb and a crunchy crust, making them ideal for serving with butter or alongside main dishes.

Prep Time: 20 minutes (active)

Cook Time: 25 minutes

Total Time: 10-12 hours (including fermentation and proofing)

Servings: 12 rolls

Ingredients:

- 400 grams Sourdough flour
- 100 grams whole wheat flour
- 350 grams water
- 100 grams active sourdough starter
- 10 grams sea salt

Instructions:

Mix the Dough: In a large bowl, combine the Sourdough flour, whole wheat flour, water, and sourdough starter. Mix until combined, then let the dough rest for 30 minutes (autolyse).

Add Salt: After the autolyse, mix in the sea salt. Fold the dough until smooth and elastic.

Bulk Fermentation: Let the dough rise for 4-6 hours at room temperature, performing stretch-and-folds every 30 minutes for the first 2 hours.

Shaping: After bulk fermentation, divide the dough into 12 equal portions. Shape each portion into a round roll and place them on a parchment-lined baking sheet.

Proofing: Cover the rolls with a damp towel and let them proof at room temperature for 1-2 hours, or refrigerate overnight.

Preheat the Oven: Preheat the oven to 425°F (220°C).

Baking: Bake the rolls for 20-25 minutes until golden brown and firm.

Cooling: Cool the rolls on a wire rack before serving warm.

These recipes provide a wide range of sourdoughs that fit seamlessly into everyday life, from flatbreads and pizza dough for quick meals to special-occasion loaves for gatherings and celebrations.

Conclusion

Sourdough bread is more than just food. It's a symbol of sustenance, community, and tradition—a staple that has nourished humanity for thousands of years. As we've explored in this book, real sourdough, made with natural ingredients and traditional methods, has the power to heal and transform our bodies from the inside out. But the journey to health through real Sourdough is about more than just the physical benefits; it's about adopting a mindful, balanced approach to how we bake, eat, and share food.

Mindful Eating and Sourdough

In today's fast-paced world, we often rush through our meals, giving little thought to the food we're consuming or how it affects our bodies. Real sourdough invites us to slow down. The process of baking sourdough —measuring ingredients, kneading dough, waiting for the slow rise—requires patience and attention. It's a practice in mindfulness, a way to connect with the food we eat and the nourishment it provides.

When we bake and eat real sourdough mindfully, we engage our senses in the process. The feel of the dough beneath our hands, the smell of fresh

Sourdough baking in the oven, the sound of the crust cracking as it cools—all of these elements remind us to be present in the moment. And when we take the time to savor each bite of the Sourdough we've made, we honor the effort, the ingredients, and the act of nourishing ourselves.

Mindful eating is not about restriction or dieting; it's about tuning in to how food makes us feel, appreciating its flavors and textures, and listening to our bodies' hunger and fullness cues. Real Sourdough , with its slow fermentation and whole grains, offers sustained energy and nutrients, making it the perfect companion for a mindful, balanced lifestyle. By eating mindfully, we can reduce stress, improve digestion, and promote a healthier relationship with food.

Sharing the Healing Power of Sourdough

One of the greatest joys of baking sourdough is the ability to share it with others. Sourdough is a communal food, meant to be broken and shared with family, friends, and neighbors. When we bake for others, we not only nourish their bodies but also strengthen connections, foster gratitude, and spread joy.

If you've discovered the healing power of real sourdough, consider extending that gift to your community. Here are a few ways to share the magic of Sourdough -making with those around you:

Bake for Your Community: Whether it's for a family dinner, a neighborhood gathering, or a donation to a local charity, sharing your sourdough with others is a simple but powerful way to bring people together. Freshly baked Sourdough is always appreciated and can be a heartwarming gesture of care and kindness.

Host Sourdough - Making Events: Invite friends, family, or neighbors to your home for a Sourdough -making workshop. Show them how to make their own loaves, teach them about the benefits of whole grains and natural fermentation, and enjoy the experience of creating something together. Sourdough - making events can be a fun, hands-on way to connect with others and share your passion for real food.

Start a Sourdough Circle: If you enjoy baking regularly, consider starting a "Sourdough circle" in your community where you and others take turns baking for each other. This could be a weekly or monthly tradition where each member bakes a loaf to share. It's a wonderful way to build a supportive, food-focused community while ensuring that everyone gets to enjoy the benefits of real sourdough.

By spreading the joy of Sourdough-baking, you're also sharing the benefits of mindful eating and real food. It's a way to connect, nurture, and inspire others on their own journey toward better health.

A Final Reflection on the Healing Power of Real Sourdough

Baking and eating real sourdough can be a life-changing experience. It's a simple act, yet it carries the potential to transform not only our health but also our approach to food, our relationships with others, and our connection to the world around us. Through the process of kneading dough, waiting for the rise, and enjoying the fruits of your labor, you learn patience, appreciation, and mindfulness.

Real sourdough teaches us that the best things in life are often the simplest—whole grains, water, salt, time, and love. When we choose real sourdough over processed, convenience-based alternatives, we're choosing to prioritize our health, our well-being, and the well-being of our communities. We're choosing to slow down, to savor, and to reconnect with what truly matters.

The journey toward health through real sourdough is an ongoing one. It's not about perfection but about progress—learning, experimenting, and enjoying the process of making and sharing food. I invite you to continue this journey with curiosity and passion. Bake often, eat mindfully, and share your sourdough with others. In doing so, you'll nourish not only your body but also your soul, cultivating a sense of well-being that radiates through every aspect of your life.

As you move forward, may real sourdough continue to be a source of strength, healing, and joy in your life. Thank you for joining me on this journey—here's to a healthier, stronger, and more vibrant you.

Index

Acknowledgements

Writing this book has been a journey of discovery, learning, and connection, and I am deeply grateful to everyone who helped make it possible. First and foremost, I would like to thank my family for their constant support and encouragement. Your patience and belief in this project kept me motivated through countless loaves of sourdough bread and many late nights.

A special thank you to the farmers and millers who preserve the tradition of growing and processing heritage grains. Your dedication to sustainable agriculture and high-quality ingredients inspired many of the recipes in this book, and your work is the foundation upon which real sourdough bread is built.

To the community of bakers, sourdough bread enthusiasts, and friends who shared their insights and experiences with me—thank you. Your passion for real sourdough and your willingness to exchange ideas have enriched this book beyond measure. It is through our collective commitment to nourishing ourselves and others that the power of real sourdough truly comes alive.

I am also grateful to my editor and publishing team for helping bring this book to life. Your thoughtful feedback and careful attention to detail have made this work clearer, more accessible, and, I hope, more impactful.

Lastly, thank you to the readers. Whether you are a seasoned baker or just beginning your journey with real sourdough bread, your interest in this book is a testament to your commitment to health and wellness. I hope that these pages inspire you to bake, to share, and to experience the healing power of real sourdough bread in your own life.